CRASH COURSE ON CHEESES

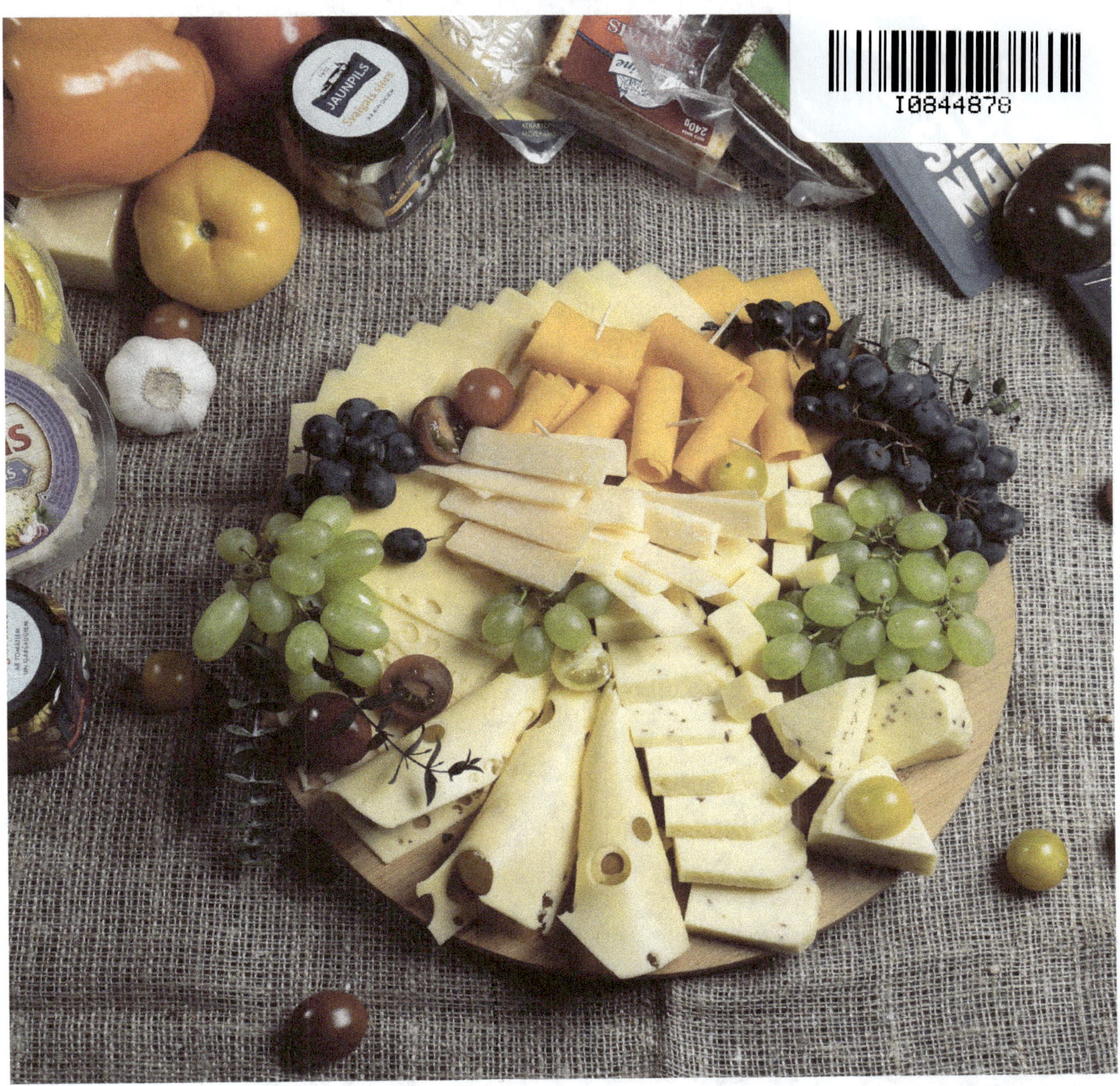

CHEESE - MILK'S LEAP TOWARD IMMORTALITY.

Cheddar

Characteristics: Cheddar is a semi-hard cheese with a pale to deep orange color, depending on the use of annatto dye. It has a creamy texture when young and becomes crumbly as it ages. The flavor ranges from mild to extra sharp, with nutty notes.

Distinguishing Feature: Cheddar's aging process significantly impacts its texture and flavor, with longer aging resulting in sharper taste and crumblier texture.

History: Cheddar originated in the English village of Cheddar in the 12th century. It has since become one of the most popular cheeses worldwide.

Prominent Use: Cheddar is used prominently in sandwiches, burgers, macaroni and cheese, and as a versatile melting cheese in various cuisines, including American and British.

Swiss (Emmental)

Characteristics: Swiss cheese is pale yellow with a sweet, nutty flavor and a firm yet slightly elastic texture. It's famous for its characteristic holes or "eyes."

Distinguishing Feature: The holes in Swiss cheese, known as "eyes," are created when carbon dioxide gas produced by bacteria gets trapped during the cheese's fermentation process.

History: Swiss cheese has a long history dating back to the Emmental region of Switzerland in the 13th century.

Prominent Use: Swiss cheese is an essential ingredient in fondue and is often used in sandwiches, particularly in the classic Reuben sandwich.

Mozzarella

Characteristics: Mozzarella is a soft, fresh cheese with a delicate milky flavor and a smooth, slightly elastic texture. It's known for its excellent melting properties.

Distinguishing Feature: Authentic buffalo mozzarella, made from water buffalo milk, is highly prized for its richer flavor and is used in traditional Italian dishes.

History: Mozzarella cheese has been made in Italy for centuries and is a key component in Neapolitan pizza.

Prominent Use: Mozzarella is widely used in Italian cuisine, especially on pizzas and in dishes like Caprese salad. It's also a popular choice for lasagna and various pasta dishes.

Brie

Characteristics: Brie is a creamy, soft cheese with a white, edible rind. Its flavor is mild, buttery, and slightly earthy, with a rich, creamy texture.

Distinguishing Feature: Brie's rind is covered in edible white mold, which contributes to its unique flavor and texture.

History: Brie de Meaux, one of the most famous varieties, has been produced in the Meaux region of France since the eighth century.

Prominent Use: Brie is often served as an appetizer with fruits, crackers, and baguettes. It can also be used in sandwiches and melted in various dishes.

Blue Cheese (e.g., Roquefort, Gorgonzola, Stilton)

Characteristics: Blue cheeses are characterized by blue-green veins of mold throughout. They have a strong, tangy flavor and a crumbly texture.

Distinguishing Feature: The blue veins are created by introducing specific Penicillium molds during the cheese-making process.

History: Roquefort, Gorgonzola, and Stilton are some of the world's oldest blue cheeses, each with a rich history and unique production methods.

Prominent Use: Blue cheeses are often used in salads, dressings, and cheese plates. They also add depth of flavor to sauces, such as Gorgonzola sauce for pasta and steak.

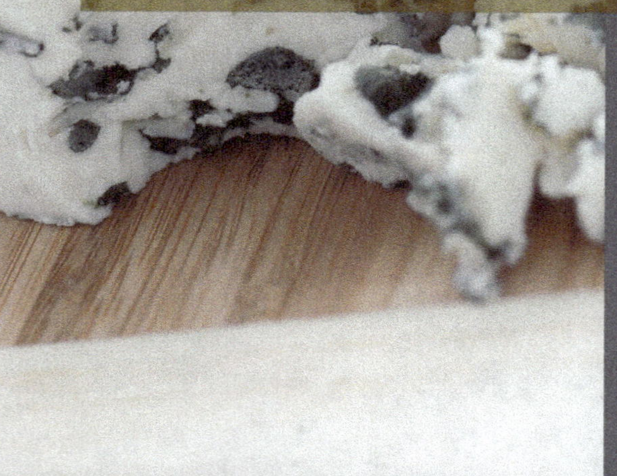

Parmesan

Characteristics: Parmesan is a hard, granular cheese with a salty, savory flavor. It's aged for at least two years, resulting in its intense flavor and granulated texture.

Distinguishing Feature: Authentic Parmesan cheese, known as Parmigiano-Reggiano, is produced in specific regions of Italy under strict regulations.

History: Parmesan cheese has been made in Italy for over 900 years and is deeply rooted in Italian culinary traditions.

Prominent Use: Parmesan is widely grated and used as a topping for pasta dishes, soups, and salads. It's a key ingredient in classic Italian dishes like risotto and eggplant Parmesan.

Crash course on World Cuisines

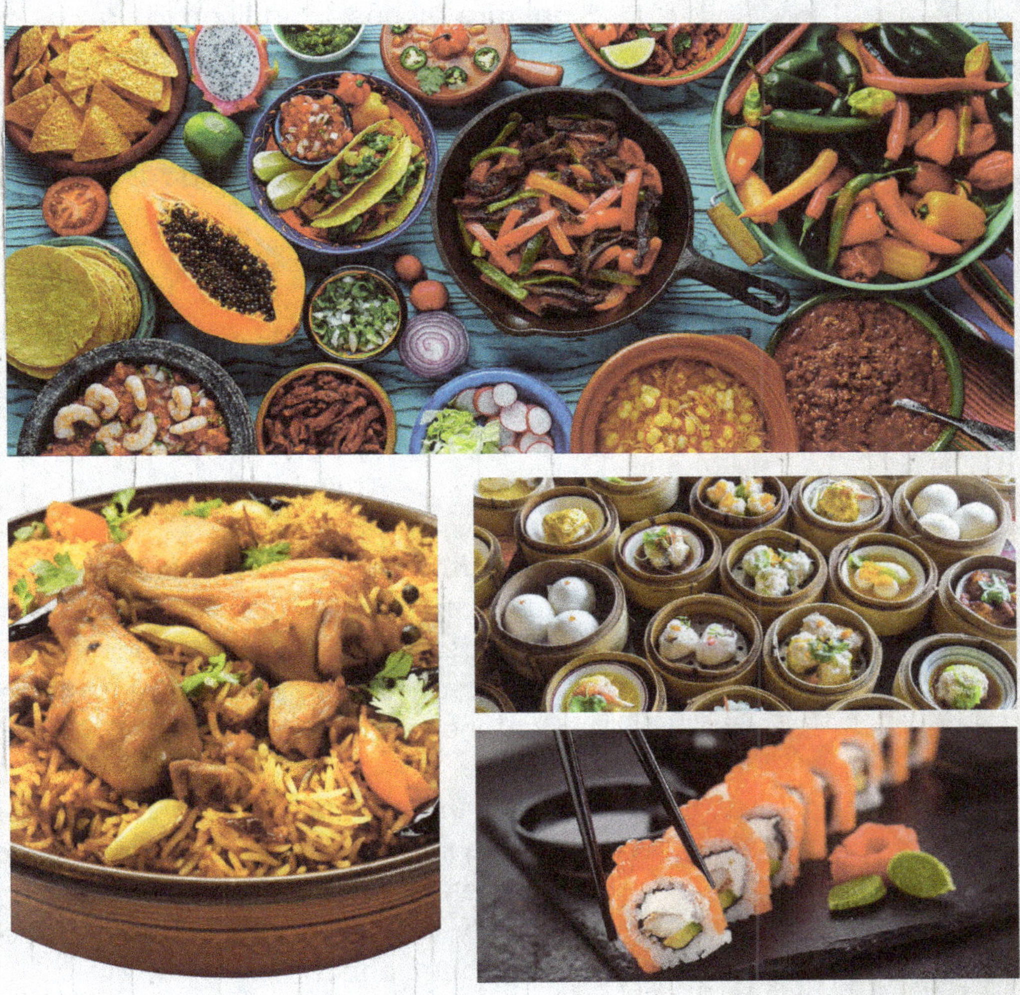

STORY OF THE WORLD READ THROUGH TASTE

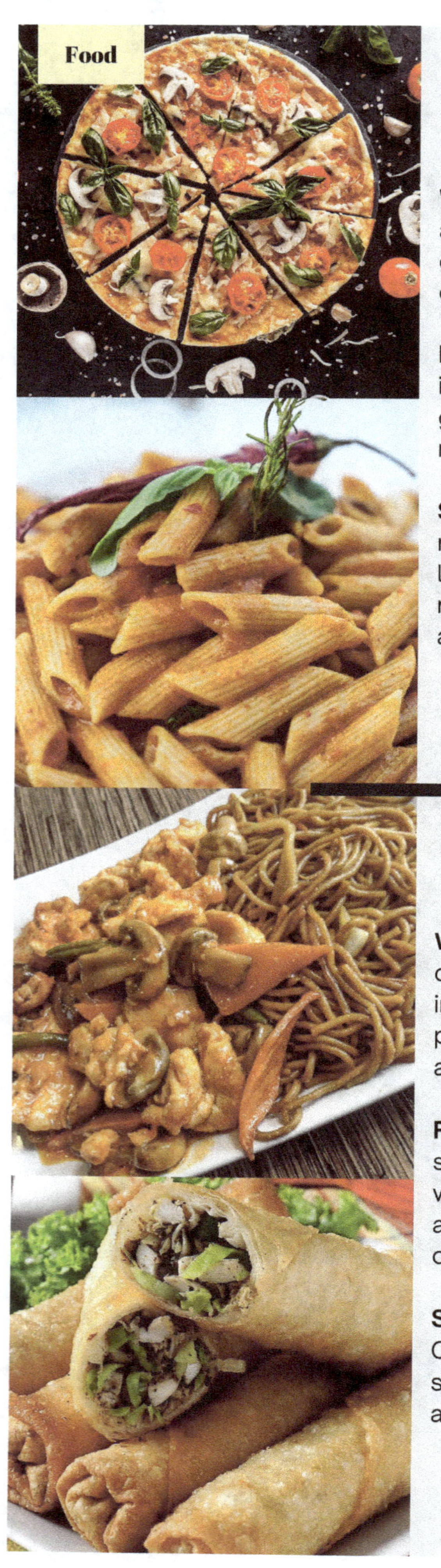

Italian Cuisine

What's Unique: Italian cuisine values simplicity and the use of high-quality, fresh ingredients. It emphasizes the natural flavors of ingredients over heavy seasoning or sauces.

Primary Ingredient: Olive oil is a fundamental ingredient in Italian cooking. Tomatoes, pasta, garlic, and a variety of cheeses like Parmesan, mozzarella, and ricotta are also central.

Signature Dishes: In addition to previously mentioned dishes, Italian cuisine boasts dishes like lasagna, gnocchi, cannoli, and various regional specialties such as Neapolitan pizza and Florentine steak (bistecca alla fiorentina).

Chinese Cuisine

What's Unique: Chinese cuisine is incredibly diverse, offering a wide range of flavors and ingredients. Regional variations are pronounced, resulting in different styles such as Cantonese, Sichuan, and Hunan.

Primary Ingredient: Rice and noodles are staples, while soy sauce, ginger, garlic, and vegetables like bok choy and Chinese broccoli are widely used. Protein sources include pork, chicken, beef, and tofu.

Signature Dishes: Beyond the classics, Chinese cuisine includes dishes like sweet and sour chicken, Peking-style duck, ma po tofu, and xiao long bao (soup dumplings).

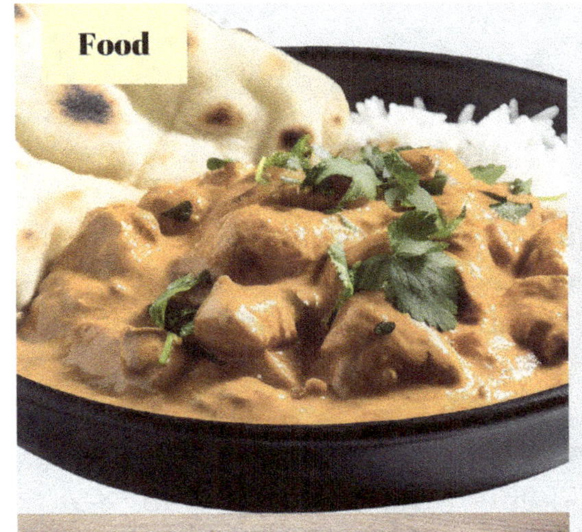

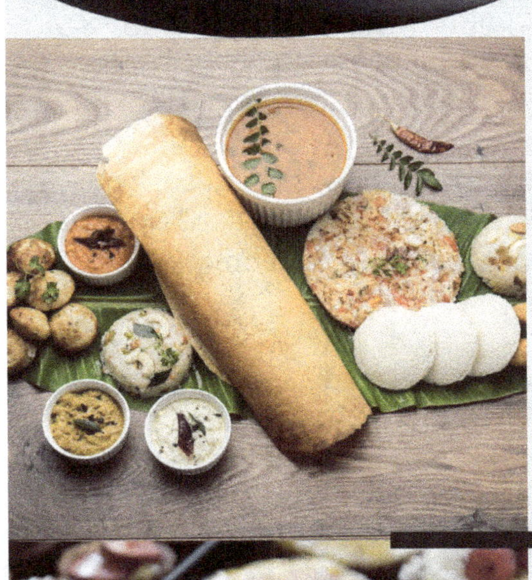

Indian Cuisine

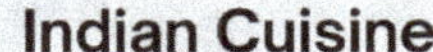

What's Unique: Indian cuisine is known for its intricate use of spices and herbs, creating layers of flavor. It offers a diverse array of vegetarian and non-vegetarian options.

Primary Ingredient: Spices like turmeric, cardamom, and cumin are essential, along with lentils, rice, and vegetables. Protein sources include chicken, lamb, and fish.

Signature Dishes: In addition to the mentioned dishes, Indian cuisine features dishes like paneer tikka, dal makhani, aloo paratha, and dosa.

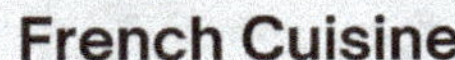

French Cuisine

What's Unique: French cuisine is celebrated for its culinary techniques, including sauces like béchamel and hollandaise. It often pairs food with wine to enhance the dining experience.

Primary Ingredient: Butter, cream, wine, and fresh herbs like thyme and parsley are commonly used. French cuisine includes proteins like duck, rabbit, and seafood.

Signature Dishes: French cuisine offers dishes like coq au vin, bouillabaisse, quiche Lorraine, and crème brûlée.

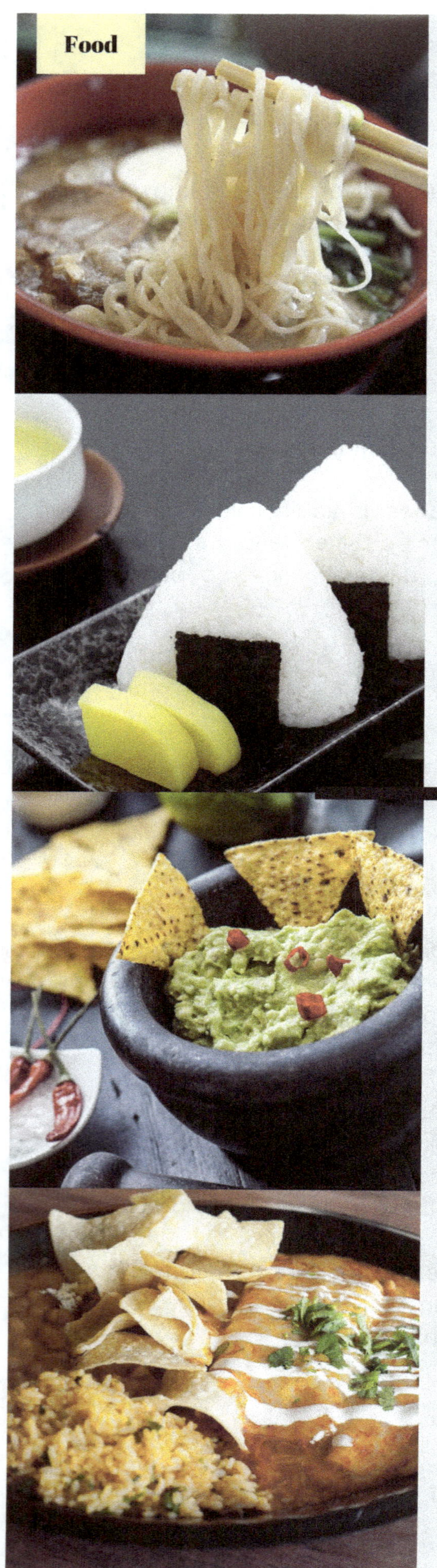

Japanese Cuisine

What's Unique: Japanese cuisine values simplicity, seasonality, and presentation. It emphasizes the natural flavors of ingredients and aesthetics.

Primary Ingredient: Rice, seafood, and seaweed are central to Japanese cooking. Soy sauce, miso, and wasabi are common condiments. Sushi-grade fish is prized.

Signature Dishes: Beyond sushi and sashimi, Japanese cuisine features dishes like tempura, yakitori, udon noodles, and okonomiyaki (savory pancake).

Mexican Cuisine

What's Unique: Mexican cuisine is known for bold and spicy flavors, often derived from chili peppers. It also features a rich combination of indigenous and Spanish influences.

Primary Ingredient: Corn, chili peppers, beans, tomatoes, and avocados are fundamental. Meats such as pork and beef are used extensively.

Signature Dishes: Mexican cuisine includes dishes like pozole, chiles en nogada, mole poblano, and elote (grilled corn on the cob).

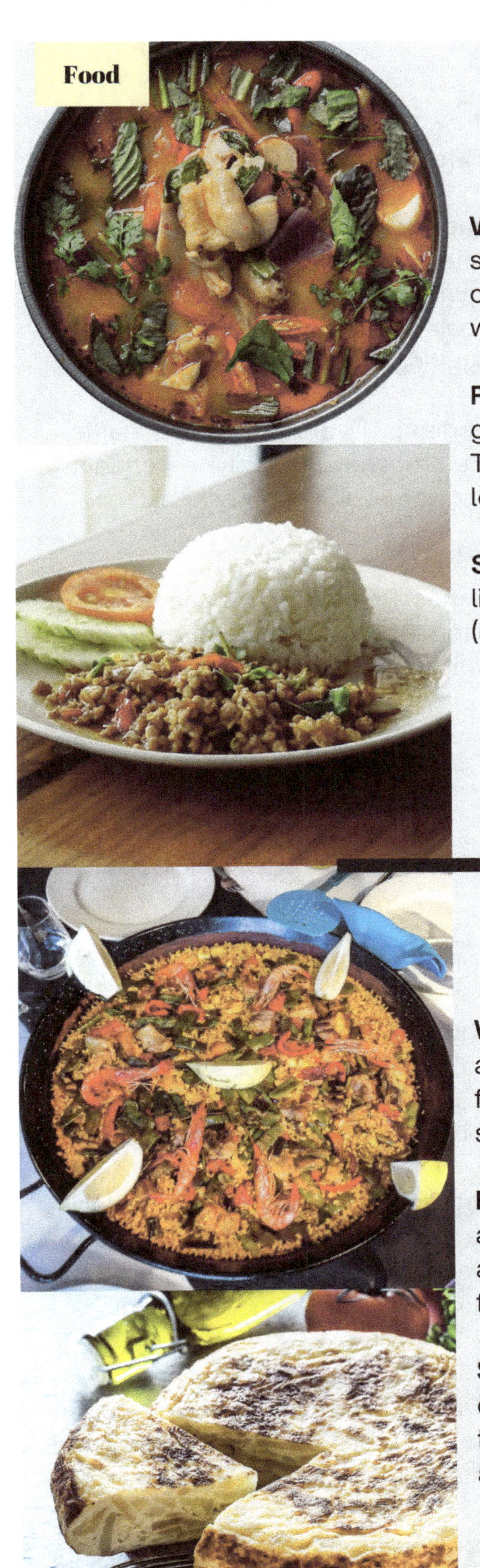

Thai Cuisine

What's Unique: Thai cuisine balances sweet, sour, salty, and spicy flavors with an emphasis on aromatic herbs and coconut milk. It offers a wide range of flavors and textures.

Primary Ingredient: Coconut milk, lemongrass, galangal, and fish sauce are key components. Thai cuisine includes ingredients like kaffir lime leaves and Thai bird's eye chilies.

Signature Dishes: Thai cuisine includes dishes like pad see ew, green curry, papaya salad (som tum), and mango sticky rice.

Spanish Cuisine

What's Unique: Spanish cuisine is diverse, with a strong focus on regional variations. It is known for bold flavors and saffron-infused rice dishes, such as paella.

Primary Ingredient: Olive oil, saffron, paprika, and various seafood like shrimp and octopus are commonly used. Spanish cuisine also features cured meats like jamón ibérico.

Signature Dishes: Spanish cuisine includes dishes like gazpacho, churros with chocolate, tapas (such as patatas bravas), and fabada asturiana (bean stew).

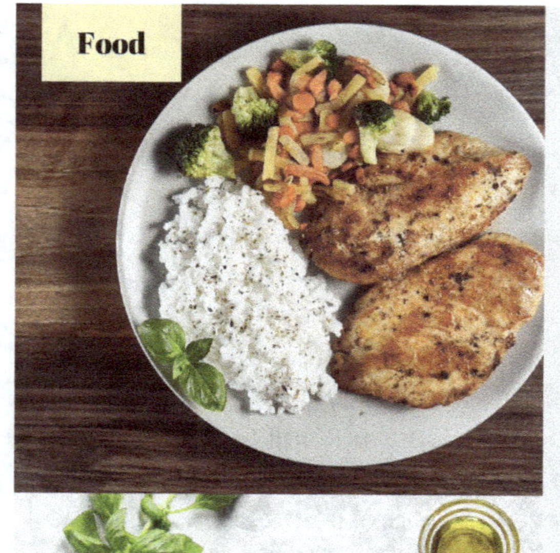

Mediterranean Cuisine

What's Unique: Mediterranean cuisine emphasizes heart-healthy ingredients like olive oil, whole grains, and fresh vegetables. It promotes a balanced and health-conscious approach to eating.

Primary Ingredient: Olive oil, tomatoes, garlic, and herbs like oregano and basil are frequently used. Seafood, lamb, and yogurt are also common.

Signature Dishes: Beyond the mentioned dishes, Mediterranean cuisine features dishes like tabbouleh, kebabs, baklava, and Greek moussaka.

.

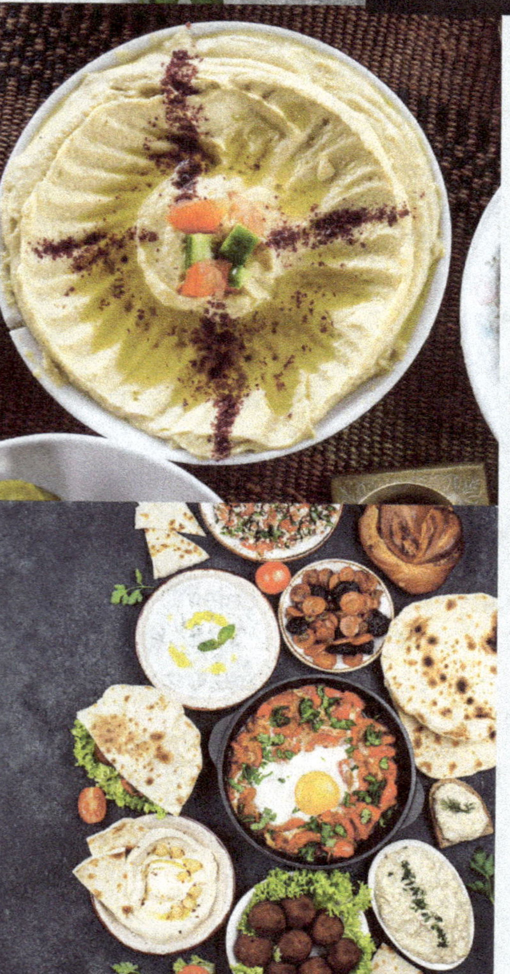

Middle Eastern Cuisine

What's Unique: Middle Eastern cuisine is characterized by aromatic spices, herbs, and a combination of sweet and savory flavors. It offers a variety of vegetarian options.

Primary Ingredient: Olive oil, tahini, pomegranate molasses, and spices like cumin, coriander, and sumac are fundamental. Ingredients like chickpeas and eggplants are common.

Signature Dishes: Middle Eastern cuisine includes dishes like shawarma, fattoush salad, baklava, and falafel.

CRASH COURSE ON BEER

Camaraderie: The sense of friendship and togetherness that comes from sharing a beer with friends, often accompanied by laughter and good conversation.

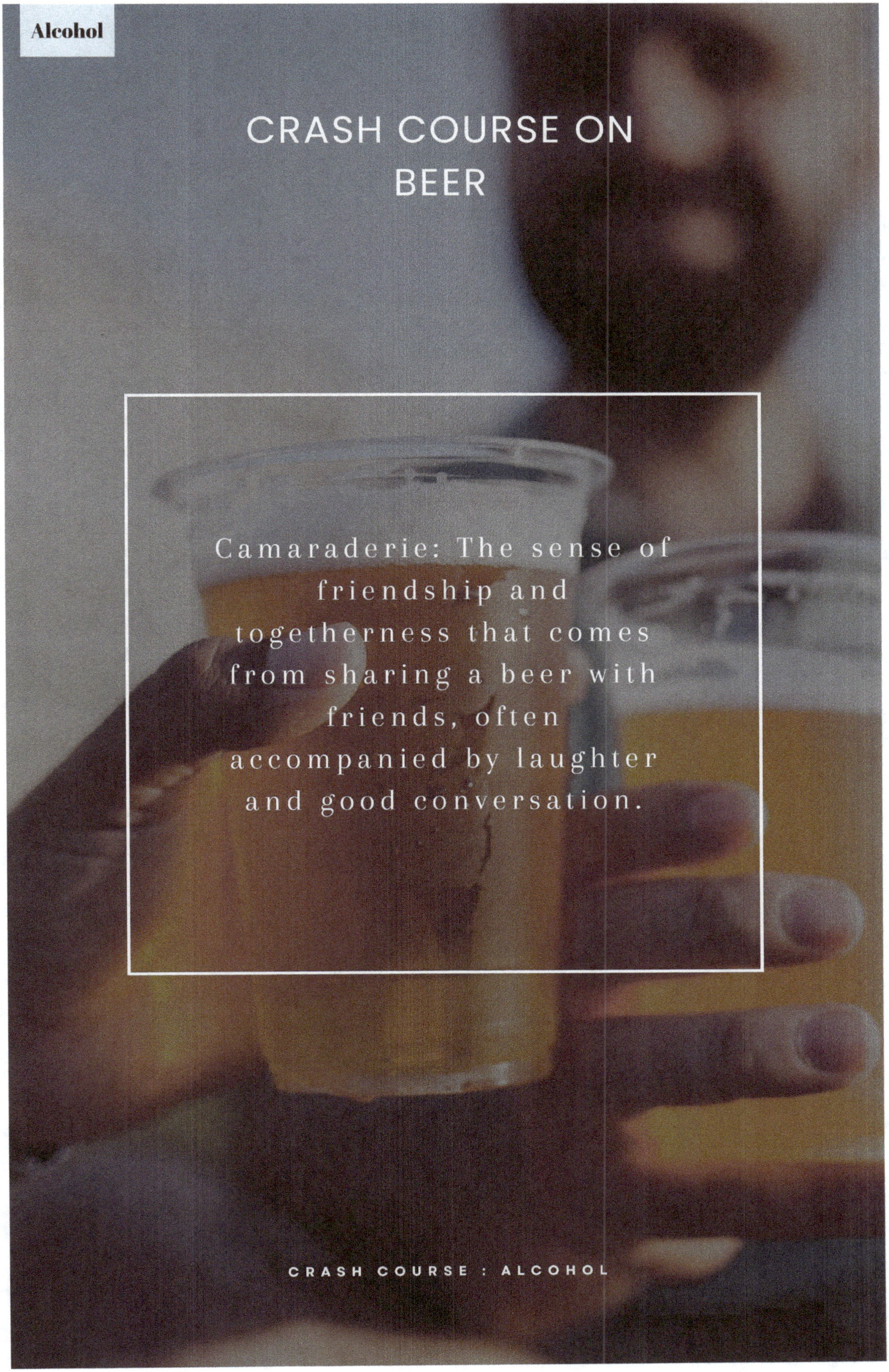

Pilsner

- **Country of Origin:** Czech Republic
- **Primary Ingredient:** Malted barley
- **Taste Characteristics:** Crisp and refreshing with a balanced bitterness, light straw to golden color, and a noticeable hop aroma.
- **Interesting Facts:** Pilsner is named after the city of Pilsen in the Czech Republic, where it was first brewed in 1842. It is one of the most popular beer styles worldwide and the inspiration for many other lager beers.

IPA (Indian Pale Ale)

- **Country of Origin:** England (although American IPAs are very popular)
- **Primary Ingredient:** Hops
- **Taste Characteristics:** Typically hoppy, with varying levels of bitterness, often with floral, citrus, or piney notes. Can range from golden to amber in color.
- **Interesting Facts:** IPAs gained popularity during the British Empire as a hoppier and higher-alcohol beer style designed to survive the long journey from England to India. American craft breweries have put their own spin on this style, leading to a wide range of IPA variations.

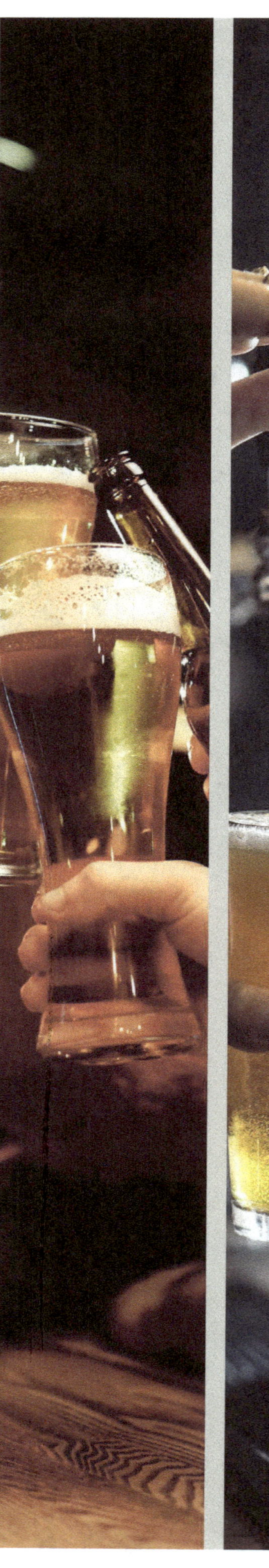
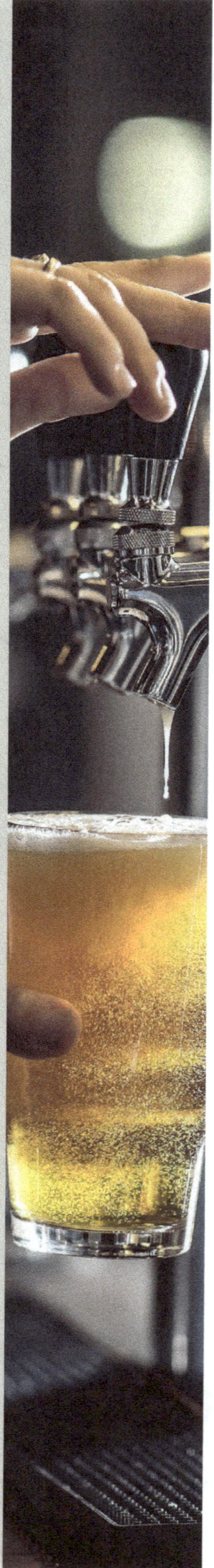

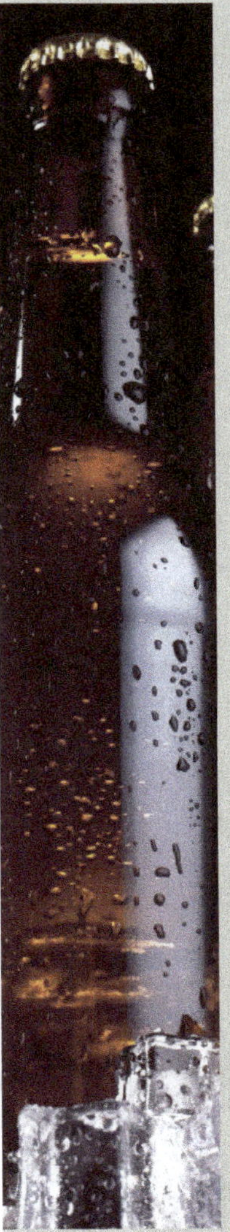

Weissbier (Hefeweizen)

- **Country of Origin:** Germany
- **Primary Ingredient:** Wheat malt
- **Taste Characteristics:** Light and refreshing with banana and clove-like flavors, cloudy appearance due to yeast, and a slightly tart finish.
- **Interesting Facts:** Weissbier is a traditional German wheat beer that is well-known for its distinctive yeast character, which gives it its unique flavor profile. It's often served with a lemon wedge in some regions.

Stout

- **Country of Origin:** Ireland (Guinness Stout) / England (Porter, which is closely related)
- **Primary Ingredient:** Roasted malted barley
- **Taste Characteristics:** Dark and rich, with flavors of coffee, chocolate, and sometimes hints of caramel. Creamy mouthfeel and often moderate bitterness.
- **Interesting Facts:** Guinness Stout, one of the most famous stouts, is known for its "cascade effect" when poured due to the use of nitrogen gas. Stout is often associated with a hearty, filling character.

Belgian Tripel

- **Country of Origin:** Belgium
- **Primary Ingredient:** A mix of malted barley and sometimes sugar
- **Taste Characteristics:** Strong and complex, with fruity, spicy, and yeasty notes. High alcohol content, often golden in color.
- **Interesting Facts:** Tripels are part of the strong ale category in Belgian beer. They are known for their deceptive drinkability despite their high alcohol content. Some famous examples include Westmalle Tripel and Chimay White.

Saison

- **Country of Origin:** Belgium / France
- **Primary Ingredient:** Pale malt and a mix of other grains
- **Taste Characteristics:** Farmhouse ales with a range of flavors, often fruity, spicy, and with a dry finish. They can vary from light to amber in color.
- **Interesting Facts:** Saisons were historically brewed in farmhouse breweries in Wallonia (Belgium) and northern France to refresh farmworkers during the summer months. They are known for their wide variety of flavor profiles.

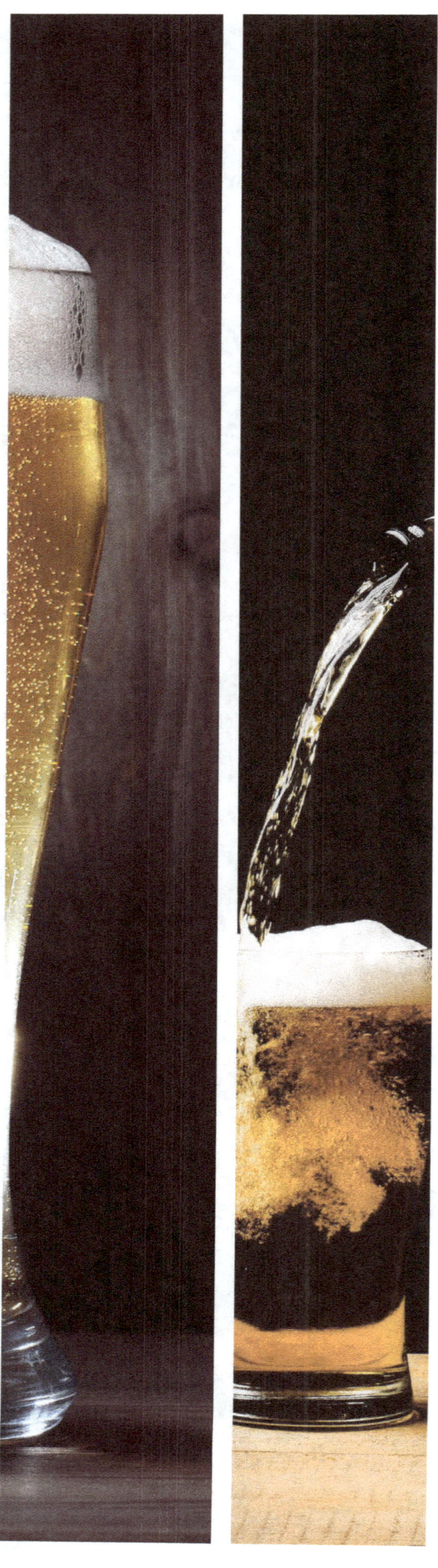

Porter

- **Country of Origin:** England
- **Primary Ingredient:** Roasted malted barley
- **Taste Characteristics:** Dark and robust, with flavors of roasted coffee, chocolate, and toffee. Often has a moderate to high bitterness level.
- **Interesting Facts:** Porter is considered one of the earliest beer styles and was a favorite of London's working class in the 18th century. It gave rise to the Stout style, and variations like the Baltic Porter are known for their richness.

Doppelbock

- **Country of Origin:** Germany
- **Primary Ingredient:** Dark malted barley
- **Taste Characteristics:** Rich and malty, with caramel and dark fruit flavors. High in alcohol content and dark brown to black in color.
- **Interesting Facts:** Doppelbock, which means "double bock," is a stronger and more robust version of the traditional German Bock beer. It was historically brewed by monks during fasting periods and is sometimes referred to as "liquid bread."

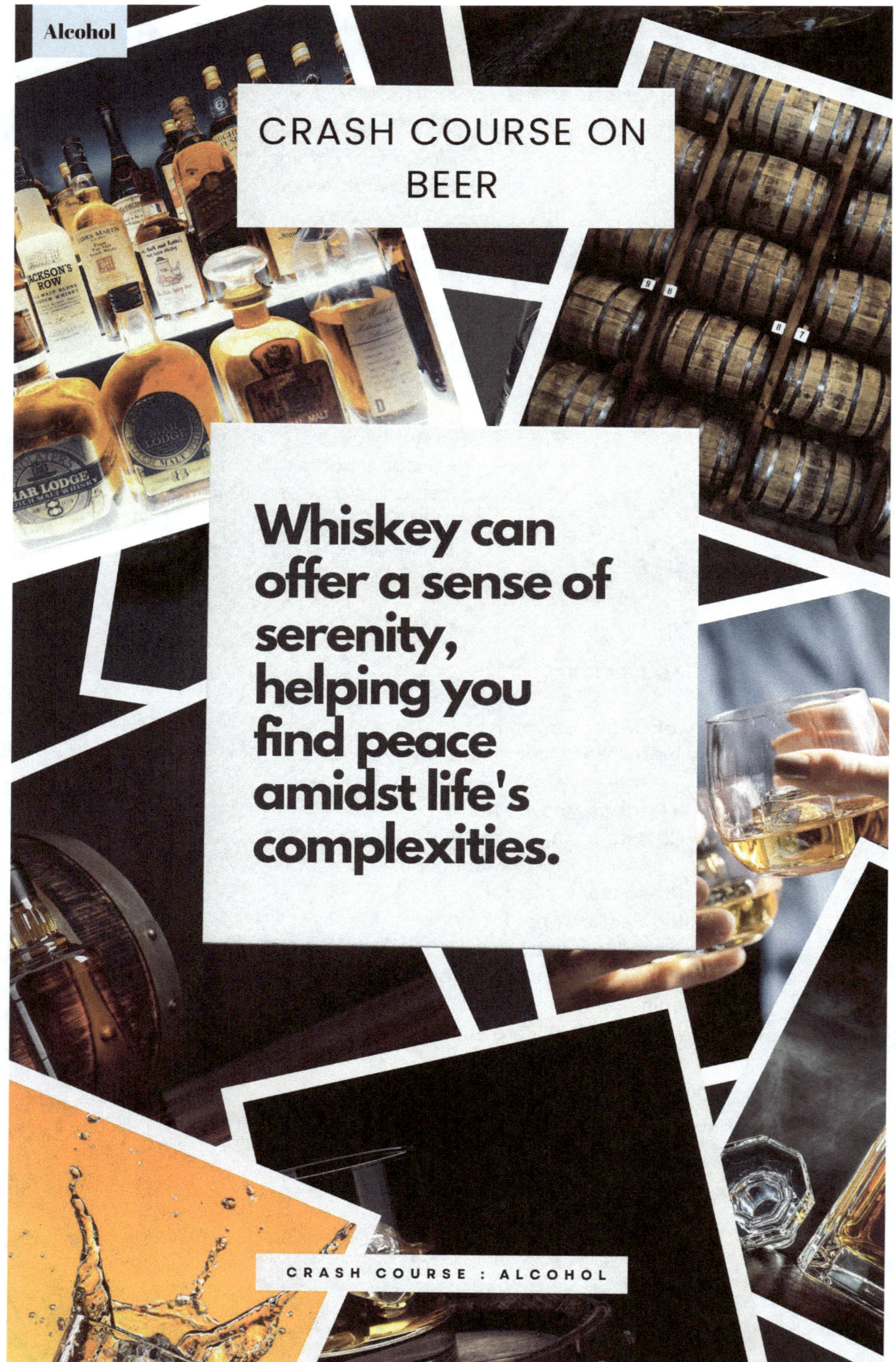
Alcohol
CRASH COURSE ON BEER
Whiskey can offer a sense of serenity, helping you find peace amidst life's complexities.
CRASH COURSE : ALCOHOL

Scotch Whisky

- **Country of Origin:** Scotland
- **Primary Ingredient:** Malted barley (although other grains can be used)
- **Taste Characteristics:** Scotch whisky can vary widely in taste, but it often has notes of peat smoke, honey, heather, and dried fruits. Single malt Scotch tends to be richer and more complex, while blended Scotch is smoother.
- **Interesting Facts:** Scotland is divided into several whisky-producing regions, each known for its unique characteristics. For example, Islay whiskies are known for their strong peaty and smoky flavors, while Speyside whiskies are often sweeter and fruitier.

Bourbon

- **Country of Origin:** United States (primarily Kentucky)
- **Primary Ingredient:** At least 51% corn (usually around 70-80%), along with malted barley and rye or wheat.
- **Taste Characteristics:** Bourbon is known for its sweet, caramel, and vanilla flavors, with hints of spice and oak. It often has a full-bodied, rich profile.
- **Interesting Facts:** Bourbon is sometimes called "America's native spirit" and must be aged in new charred oak barrels. Kentucky, particularly the region around Louisville, is famous for producing some of the world's finest bourbons.

Irish Whiskey

- **Country of Origin:** Ireland
- **Primary Ingredient:** Malted and unmalted barley (some use other grains)
- **Taste Characteristics:** Irish whiskey is typically smooth and approachable, with notes of honey, vanilla, and light fruitiness. It is known for its triple distillation process.
- **Interesting Facts:** Ireland claims to be the birthplace of whiskey, and there are many distilleries with centuries-old traditions. Irish whiskey has seen a resurgence in popularity in recent years.

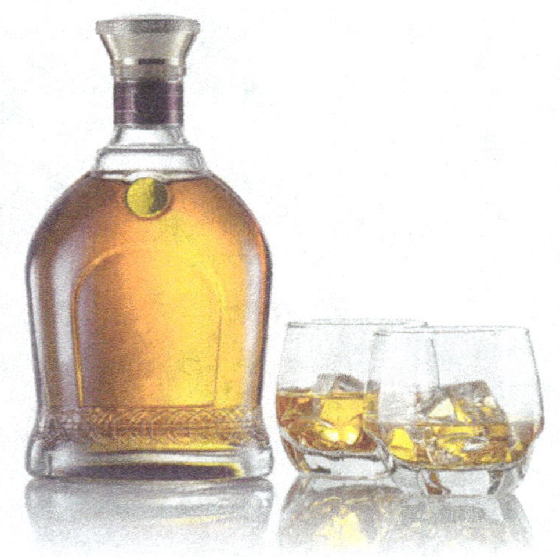

Rye Whiskey

- **Country of Origin:** United States and Canada
- **Primary Ingredient:** At least 51% rye grain (higher rye content than bourbon)
- **Taste Characteristics:** Rye whiskey tends to have a spicier and more robust flavor profile compared to bourbon, with notes of pepper, cinnamon, and sometimes fruity undertones.
- **Interesting Facts:** Rye whiskey has a rich history, with both American and Canadian variations. It was a popular choice during the pre-prohibition era and has made a comeback in craft distilleries.

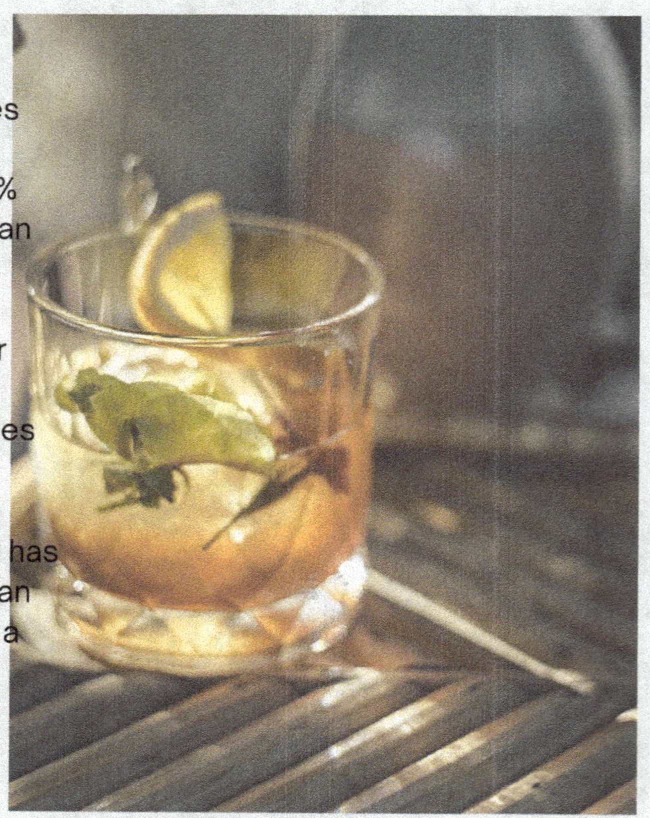

Japanese Whisky

- **Country of Origin:** Japan
- **Primary Ingredient:** Typically malted barley, although some Japanese whiskies use corn and other grains.
- **Taste Characteristics:** Japanese whisky often features a delicate and balanced flavor profile, with notes of orchard fruits, honey, and gentle oak. It's known for its craftsmanship and precision.
- **Interesting Facts:** Japanese whisky has gained international acclaim for its quality and has won numerous awards in blind tastings, challenging traditional whisky-producing regions.

Single Malt Whisky (Scotch Single Malt):

- **Ingredients:** Single malt Scotch whisky is made from 100% malted barley. It is a specific type of Scotch whisky that excludes other grains.
- **Production:** Single malt whisky is produced at a single distillery, meaning all the whisky in the bottle comes from one distillery. It is distilled in pot stills and aged in oak barrels, typically for a minimum of three years.
- **Flavor Profile:** Single malt Scotch whiskies are known for their distinct and often complex flavors, which can vary significantly depending on the distillery, region, and aging process. They may have fruity, floral, peaty, or other unique characteristics.
- **Region:** Single malt Scotch can come from various regions within Scotland, each known for its particular flavor profile. For example, Islay single malts are known for their peaty and smoky flavors, while Speyside single malts tend to be sweeter and fruitier.

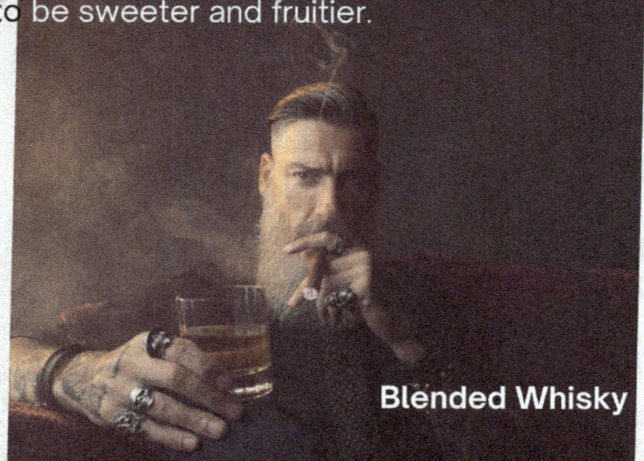

- **Ingredients:** Blended whisky is a blend of multiple whiskies, which can include malt whisky and grain whisky. Grain whisky is often made from grains like corn, wheat, or rye
- **Production:** Blended whisky is created by mixing different whiskies from various distilleries. It is a combination of malt whisky and grain whisky.
- **Aging:** The individual components of a blended whisky may have different aging periods and come from various sources. Some may be aged longer for flavor development, while others may be used to add milder characteristics.
- **Flavor Profile:** Blended whiskies are designed to have a more balanced and approachable flavor profile. They often aim to combine the complexity of malt whisky with the smoother and milder qualities of grain whisky.
- **Consistency:** Blended whiskies are known for their consistency and uniform flavor. Master blenders carefully select and blend different components to maintain a specific taste profile, ensuring that each bottle tastes very similar to the last.

Crash Course on

Gin

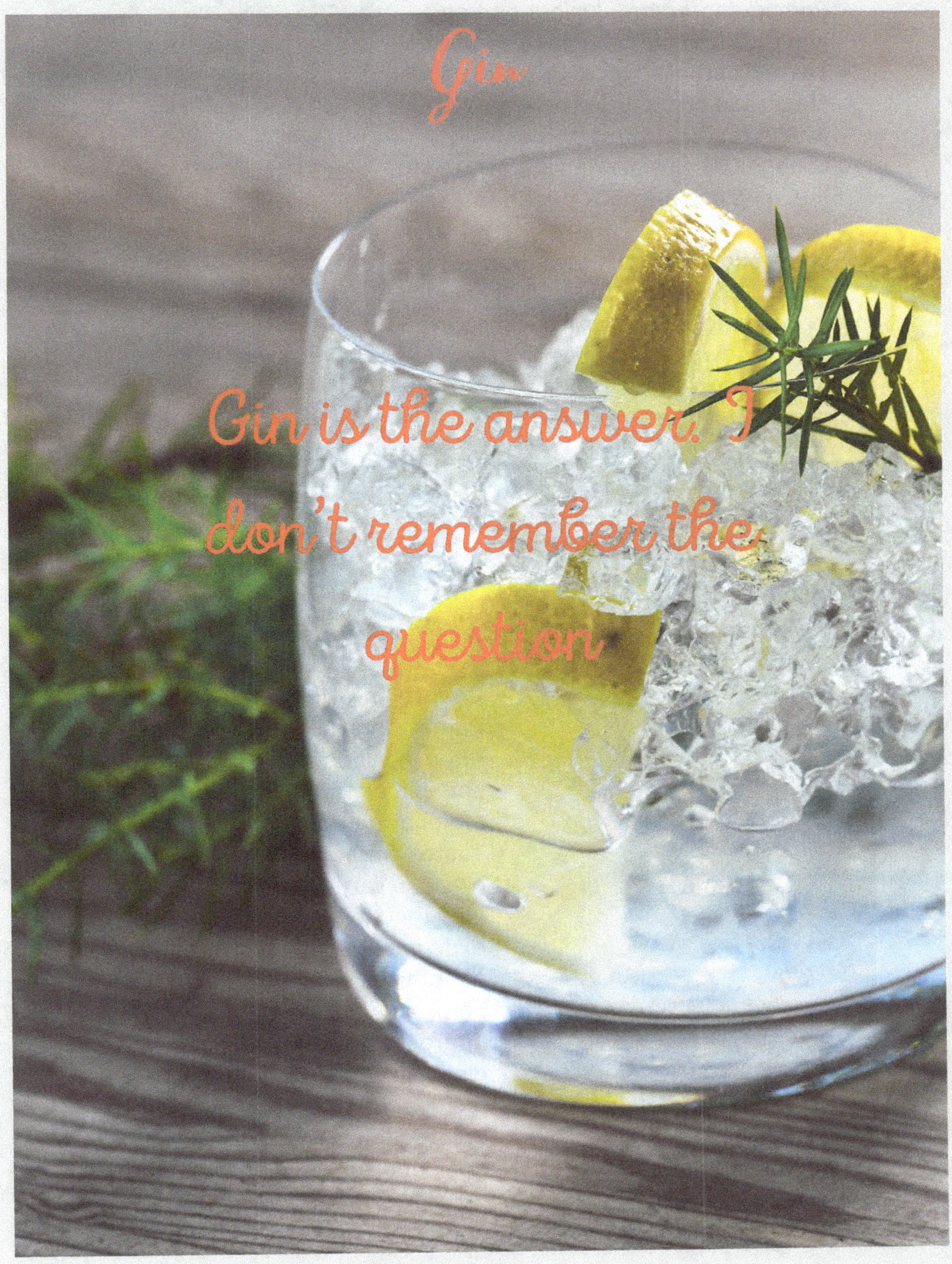

London Dry Gin

- **Country of Origin:** England
- **Primary Ingredient:** Juniper berries and a neutral grain spirit
- **Taste Characteristics:** Crisp, clean, and typically juniper-forward with herbal and citrus notes. London Dry gins are known for their dryness and lack of added sugar.
- **Interesting Facts:** Despite the name, London Dry Gin doesn't have to be made in London. It's a style of gin known for its strict production methods and botanical balance.

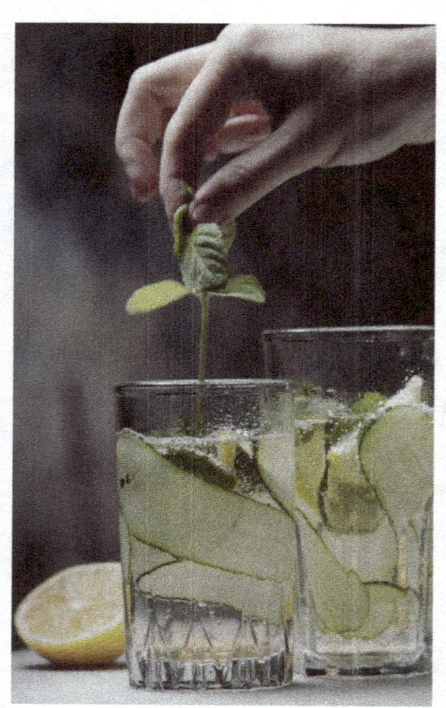

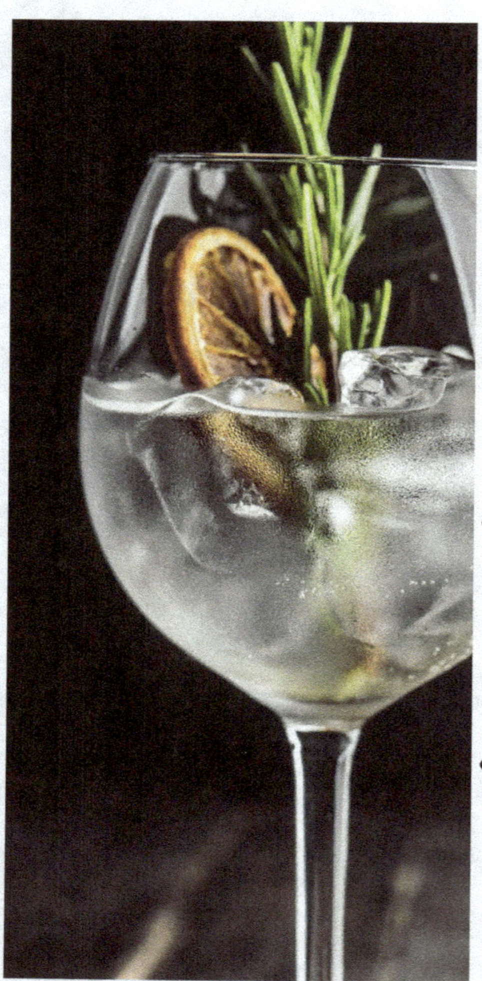

American Gin

- **Country of Origin:** United States
- **Primary Ingredient:** Varies, but often includes a mix of botanicals, sometimes with a focus on local or regional ingredients.
- **Taste Characteristics:** American gins can vary widely in flavor, but they tend to be more experimental, with a diverse range of botanicals, including citrus, herbs, and spices.
- **Interesting Facts:** American craft distilleries have contributed to a resurgence of gin production in the United States, leading to a wide array of unique and creative gins.

Old Tom Gin

- **Country of Origin:** England
- **Primary Ingredient:** Juniper berries and a slightly sweetened spirit (typically with sugar or syrup)
- **Taste Characteristics:** A bridge between the drier London Dry style and the sweeter Genever style. It has a gentle sweetness and a more rounded flavor profile.
- **Interesting Facts:** Old Tom Gin was popular in the 18th century and was traditionally served in gin cocktails like the Tom Collins.

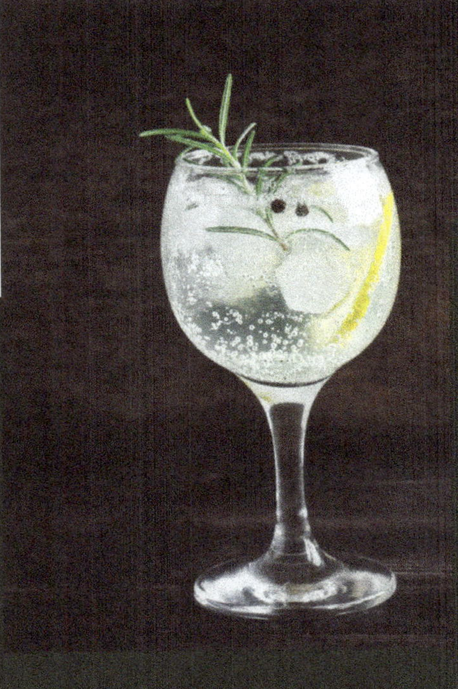

Genever

- **Country of Origin:** England
- **Primary Ingredient:** Netherlands and Belgium
- **Primary Ingredient:** Malted barley, juniper berries, and a mix of other botanicals.
- **Taste Characteristics:** Rich, malty, and often sweeter than London Dry gins. It has a grainier texture and a more pronounced juniper and herbal flavor.
- **Interesting Facts:** Genever is considered the precursor to modern gin, and it has a long history dating back to the 16th century.

Plymouth Gin

- **Country of Origin:** England (Plymouth, specifically)
- **Primary Ingredient:** Juniper berries, coriander seeds, and sweet orange peel, among other botanicals.
- **Taste Characteristics:** Smooth and slightly sweeter than London Dry gins, with a more pronounced earthy and citrusy flavor profile.
- **Interesting Facts:** Plymouth Gin has a Protected Geographical Indication (PGI) status, which means it must be made in Plymouth to be called "Plymouth Gin."

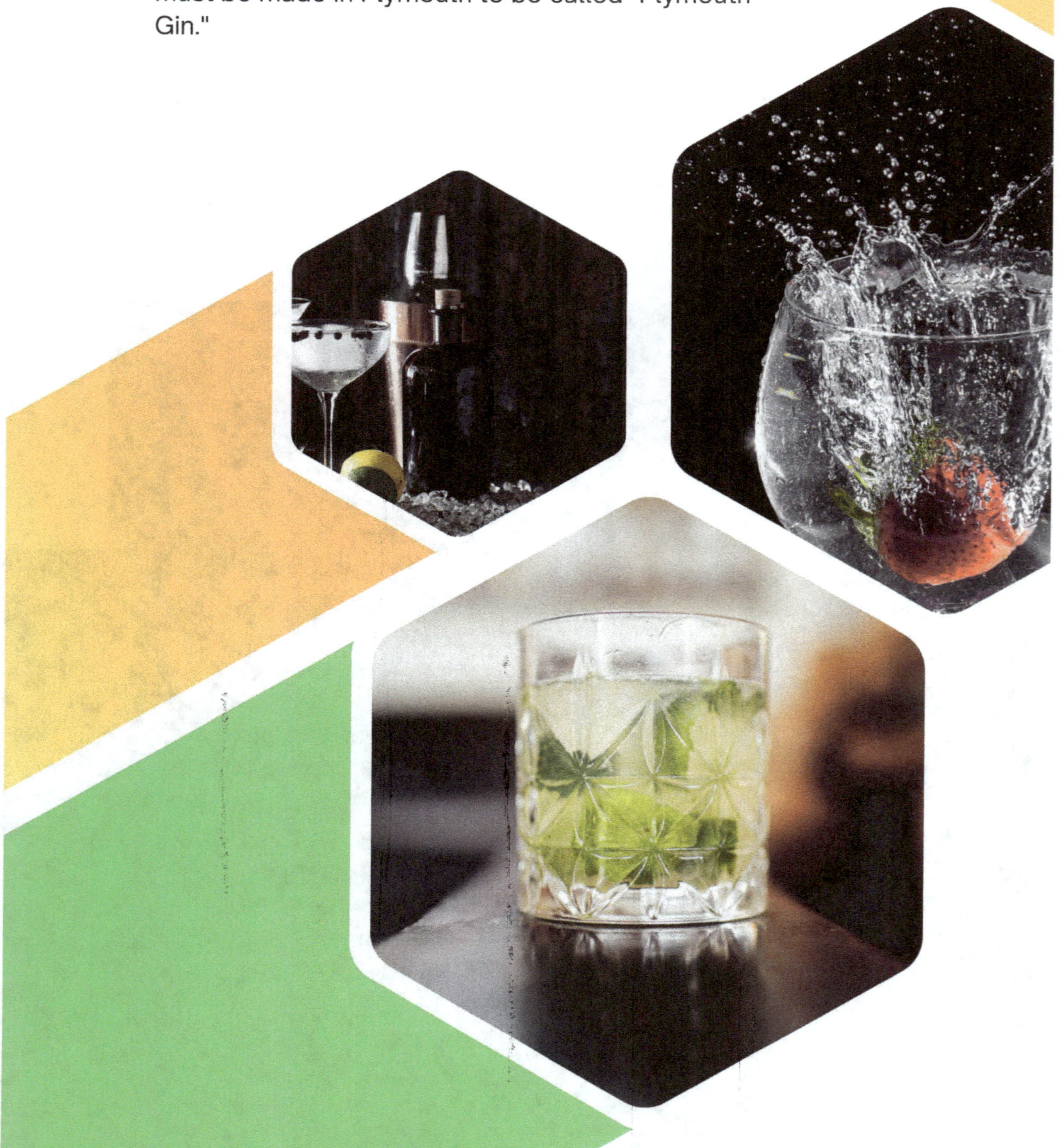

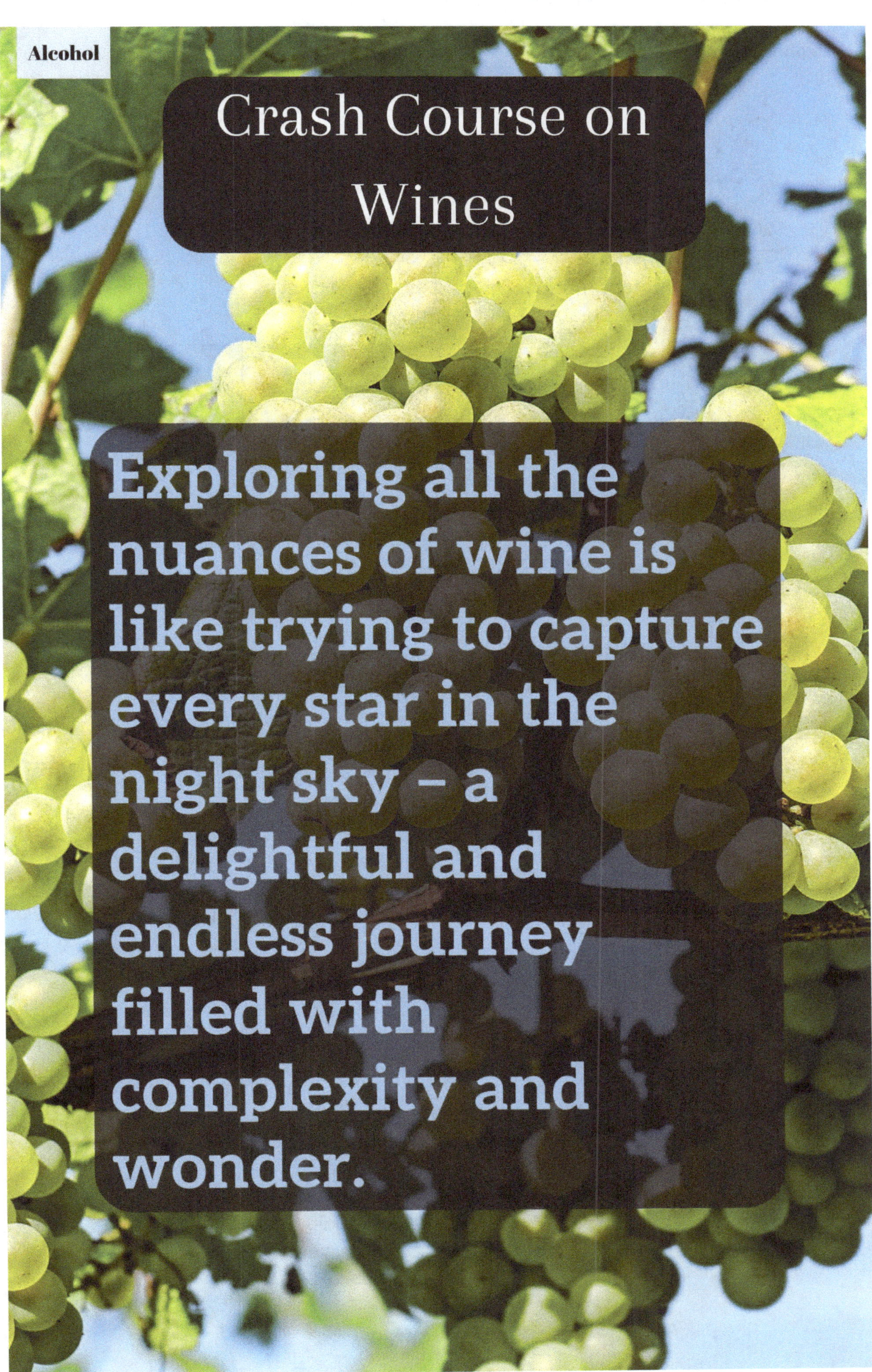
Alcohol
Crash Course on Wines
Exploring all the nuances of wine is like trying to capture every star in the night sky – a delightful and endless journey filled with complexity and wonder.

Cabernet Sauvignon

- **Country of Origin:** France (Bordeaux region)
- **Primary Ingredient:** Cabernet Sauvignon grapes
- **Taste Characteristics:** Full-bodied, with flavors of blackcurrant, plum, and sometimes hints of green bell pepper. Tannic and often aged in oak, which can add notes of vanilla and cedar.
- **Interesting Facts:** Cabernet Sauvignon is one of the world's most widely recognized and planted grape varieties. It's known for its aging potential and is often called the "King of Red Wine Grapes."

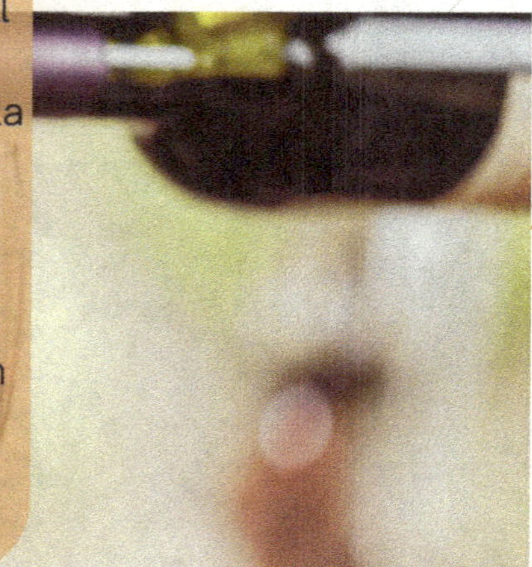

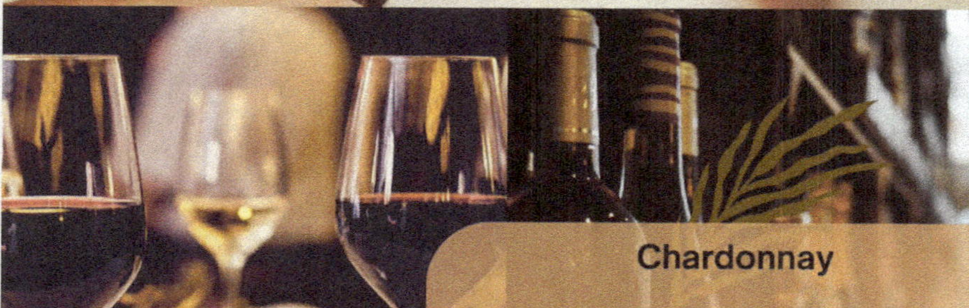

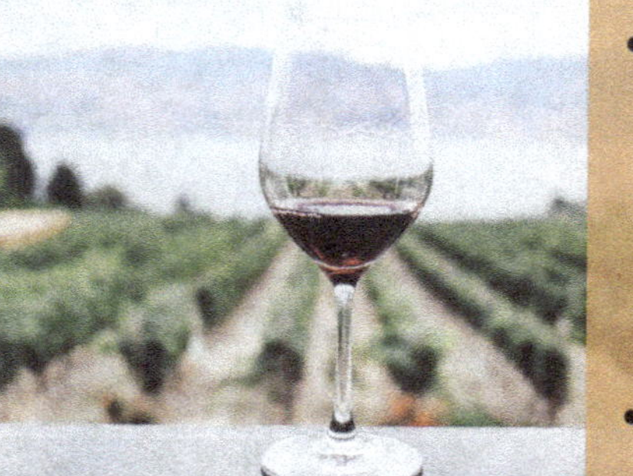

Chardonnay

- **Country of Origin:** France (Burgundy region)
- **Primary Ingredient:** Chardonnay grapes
- **Taste Characteristics:** A diverse range of flavors depending on winemaking techniques. Common notes include green apple, citrus, and buttery characteristics in oak-aged versions.
- **Interesting Facts:** Chardonnay is one of the most versatile white wine grapes. It can be used to make sparkling wine (Champagne), unoaked wines, and rich, full-bodied oaked wines.

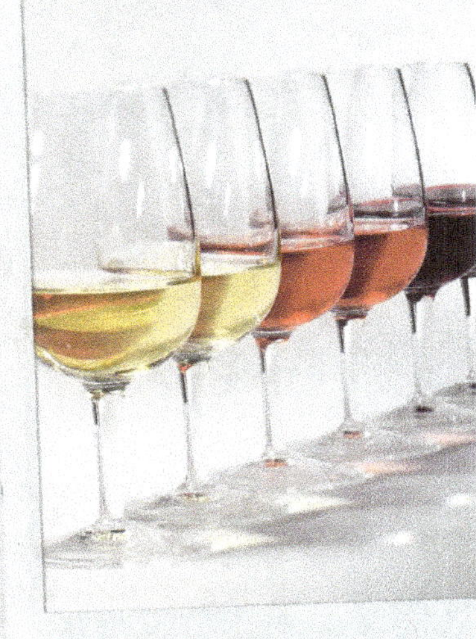

Merlot

- **Country of Origin:** France (Bordeaux region)
- **Primary Ingredient:** Merlot grapes
- **Taste Characteristics:** Soft, velvety texture with flavors of plum, cherry, and sometimes herbal notes. Generally less tannic and more approachable than Cabernet Sauvignon.
- **Interesting Facts:** Merlot is often used in Bordeaux blends but is also produced as a single varietal wine. It's known for its smooth and easy-drinking qualities.

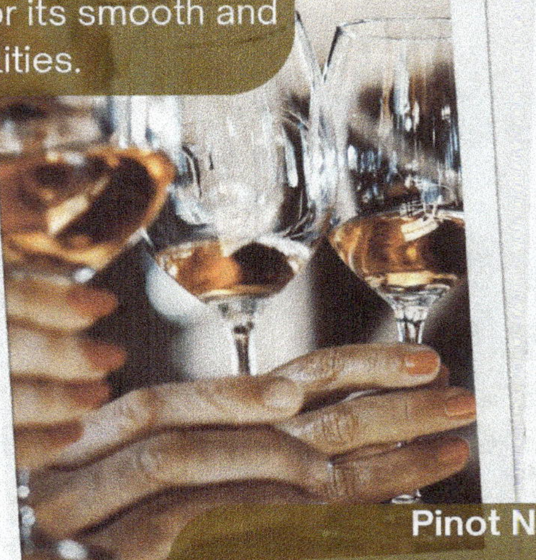

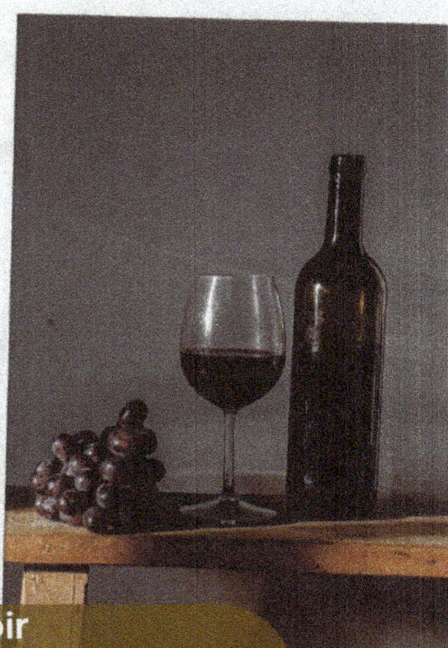

Pinot Noir

- **Country of Origin:** France (Burgundy region)
- **Primary Ingredient:** Pinot Noir grapes
- **Taste Characteristics:** Light to medium-bodied with red fruit flavors like cherry and raspberry, often with earthy or floral notes. Delicate and nuanced.
- **Interesting Facts:** Pinot Noir is notoriously difficult to cultivate and is highly sensitive to its growing environment. It's considered by many to produce some of the world's finest wines.

Sauvignon Blanc

- **Country of Origin:** France (Bordeaux and Loire Valley)
- **Primary Ingredient:** Sauvignon Blanc grapes
- **Taste Characteristics:** Crisp and refreshing with high acidity. Flavors include green apple, citrus, grass, and sometimes tropical fruit notes.
- **Interesting Facts:** Sauvignon Blanc is used to make a wide range of wines, from the zesty and herbaceous examples of the Loire Valley to the more tropical and grassy versions of New Zealand.

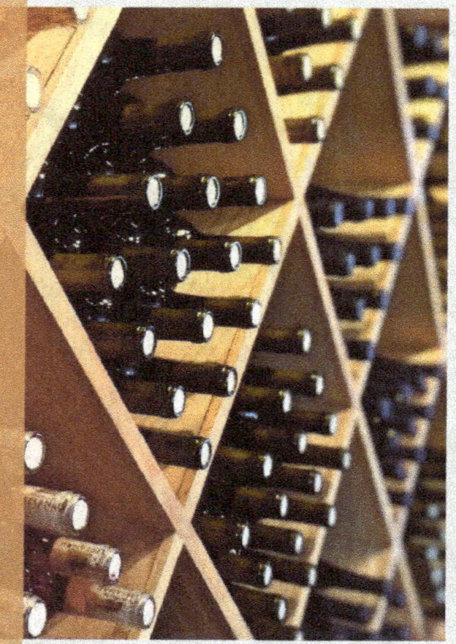

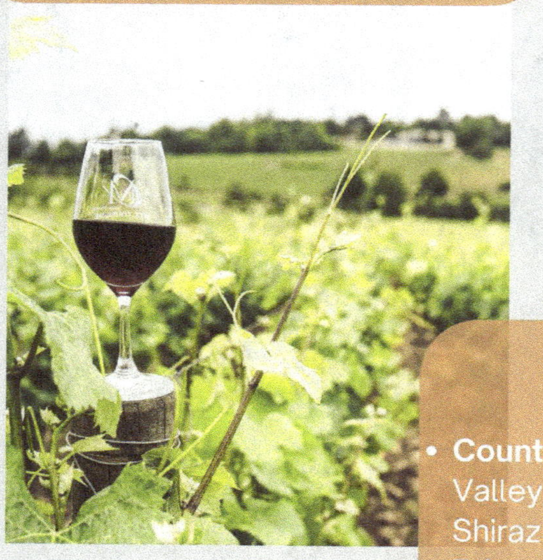

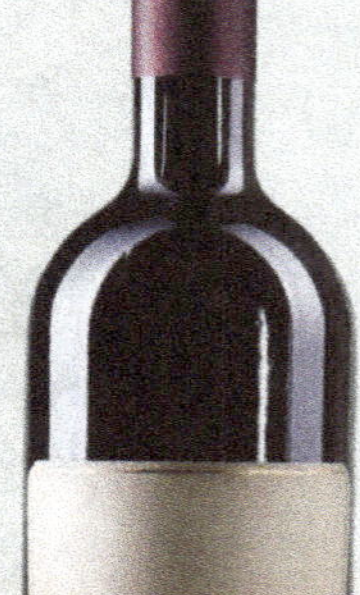

Syrah/Shiraz

- **Country of Origin:** France (Rhone Valley) for Syrah, Australia for Shiraz
- **Primary Ingredient:** Syrah/Shiraz grapes
- **Taste Characteristics:** Rich and full-bodied with flavors of blackberry, plum, black pepper, and sometimes smoked meat or spice.
- **Interesting Facts:** The grape is known as Syrah in France and Shiraz in Australia. It produces bold and intense red wines in both regions.

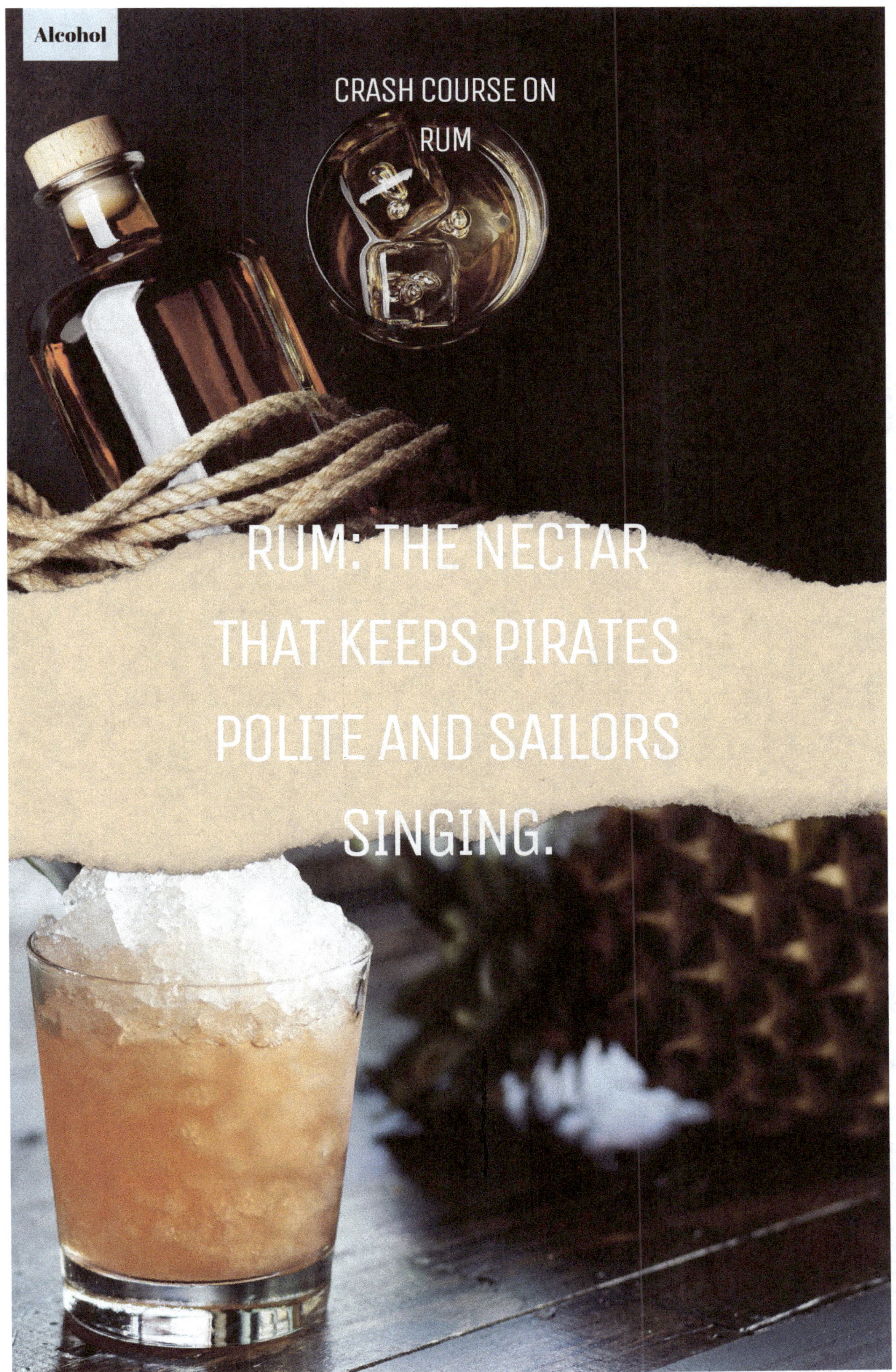
CRASH COURSE ON
RUM
RUM: THE NECTAR
THAT KEEPS PIRATES
POLITE AND SAILORS
SINGING.

Country of Origin: Caribbean

- **Primary Ingredient:** Sugarcane Juice or Molasses
- **Taste Characteristics:** Caribbean rums vary widely in flavor, but they often feature notes of tropical fruits, vanilla, caramel, and spices. Lighter rums are more delicate and sweet, while darker rums are richer and may have hints of oak and tobacco.
- **Interesting Facts:** The Caribbean is a diverse region for rum production, with countries like Jamaica, Barbados, Cuba, and Puerto Rico known for their unique rum styles. For example, Jamaican rum is famous for its funky and robust flavor due to the use of dunder and ester-rich yeast strains.

Country of Origin: Cuba

- **Primary Ingredient:** Molasses
- **Taste Characteristics:** Cuban rums are known for their smooth and light profiles, often featuring notes of vanilla, citrus, and a subtle sweetness. They are typically aged in oak barrels, imparting a mellow character.
- **Interesting Facts:** Cuba is renowned for its iconic rum cocktails, including the Mojito and the Daiquiri, both of which use Cuban rum as a key ingredient. Havana Club is one of the most famous Cuban rum brands.

Country of Origin: Jamaica

- **Primary Ingredient:** Sugarcane Juice or Molasses
- **Taste Characteristics:** Jamaican rums are known for their bold and complex flavors, often characterized by tropical fruit, banana, and funky, earthy notes. They can have a strong, pungent aroma and are sometimes referred to as "hogo" rum.
- **Interesting Facts:** Jamaican rums are distinct because of the use of pot stills and the unique fermentation process, which contributes to their robust flavor. They are frequently used in tiki cocktails due to their strong character.

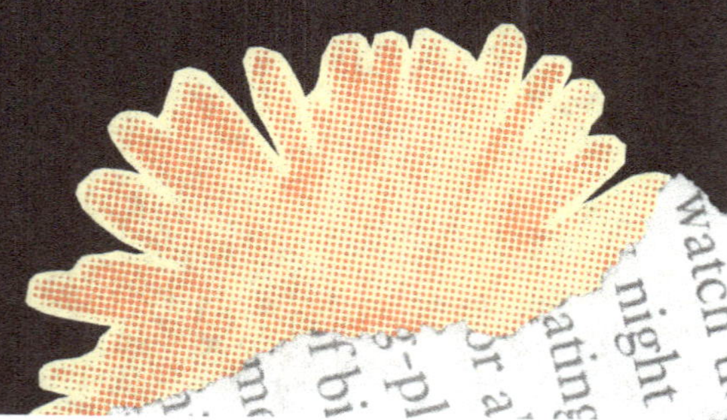

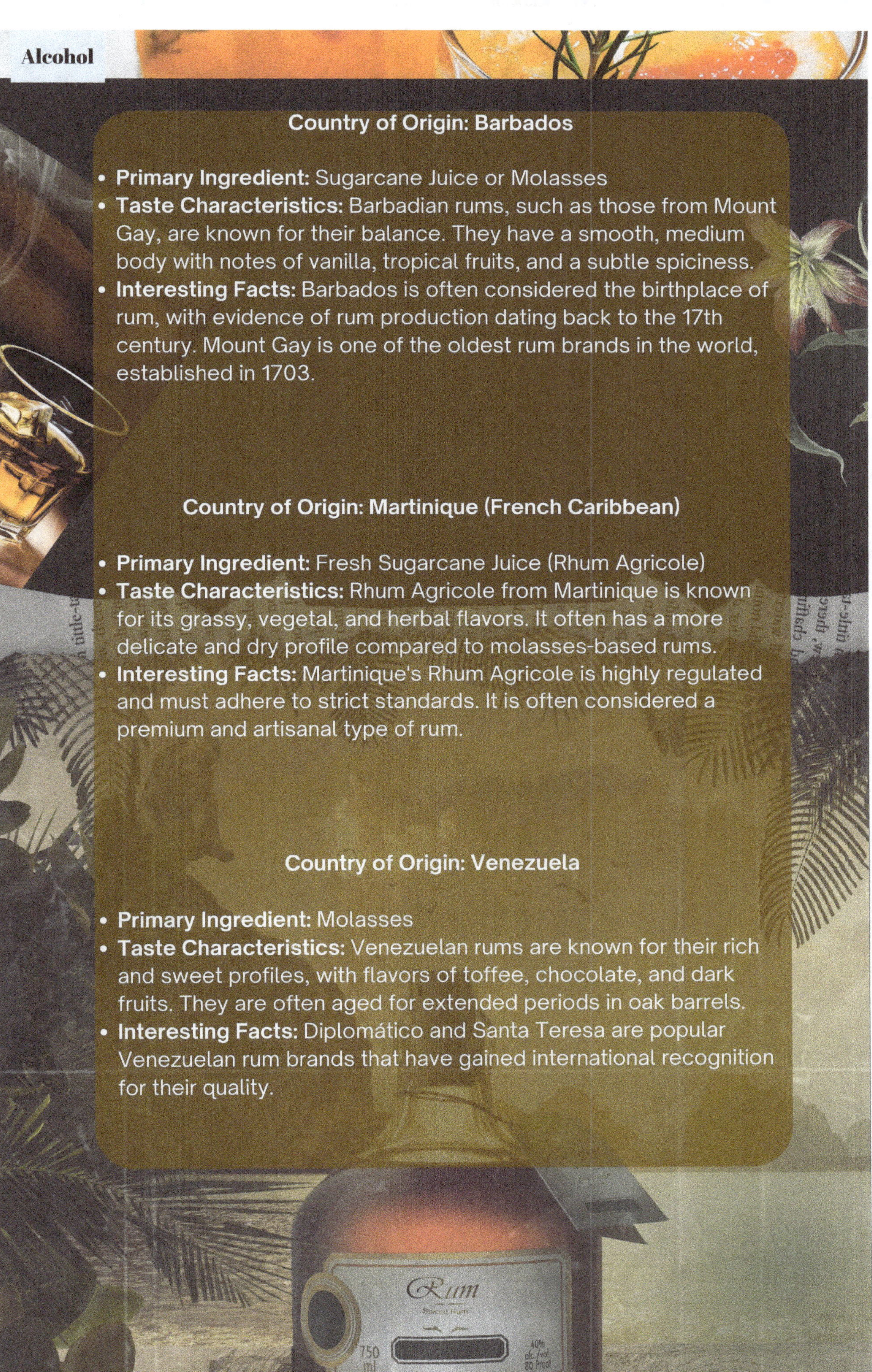

Country of Origin: Barbados

- **Primary Ingredient:** Sugarcane Juice or Molasses
- **Taste Characteristics:** Barbadian rums, such as those from Mount Gay, are known for their balance. They have a smooth, medium body with notes of vanilla, tropical fruits, and a subtle spiciness.
- **Interesting Facts:** Barbados is often considered the birthplace of rum, with evidence of rum production dating back to the 17th century. Mount Gay is one of the oldest rum brands in the world, established in 1703.

Country of Origin: Martinique (French Caribbean)

- **Primary Ingredient:** Fresh Sugarcane Juice (Rhum Agricole)
- **Taste Characteristics:** Rhum Agricole from Martinique is known for its grassy, vegetal, and herbal flavors. It often has a more delicate and dry profile compared to molasses-based rums.
- **Interesting Facts:** Martinique's Rhum Agricole is highly regulated and must adhere to strict standards. It is often considered a premium and artisanal type of rum.

Country of Origin: Venezuela

- **Primary Ingredient:** Molasses
- **Taste Characteristics:** Venezuelan rums are known for their rich and sweet profiles, with flavors of toffee, chocolate, and dark fruits. They are often aged for extended periods in oak barrels.
- **Interesting Facts:** Diplomático and Santa Teresa are popular Venezuelan rum brands that have gained international recognition for their quality.

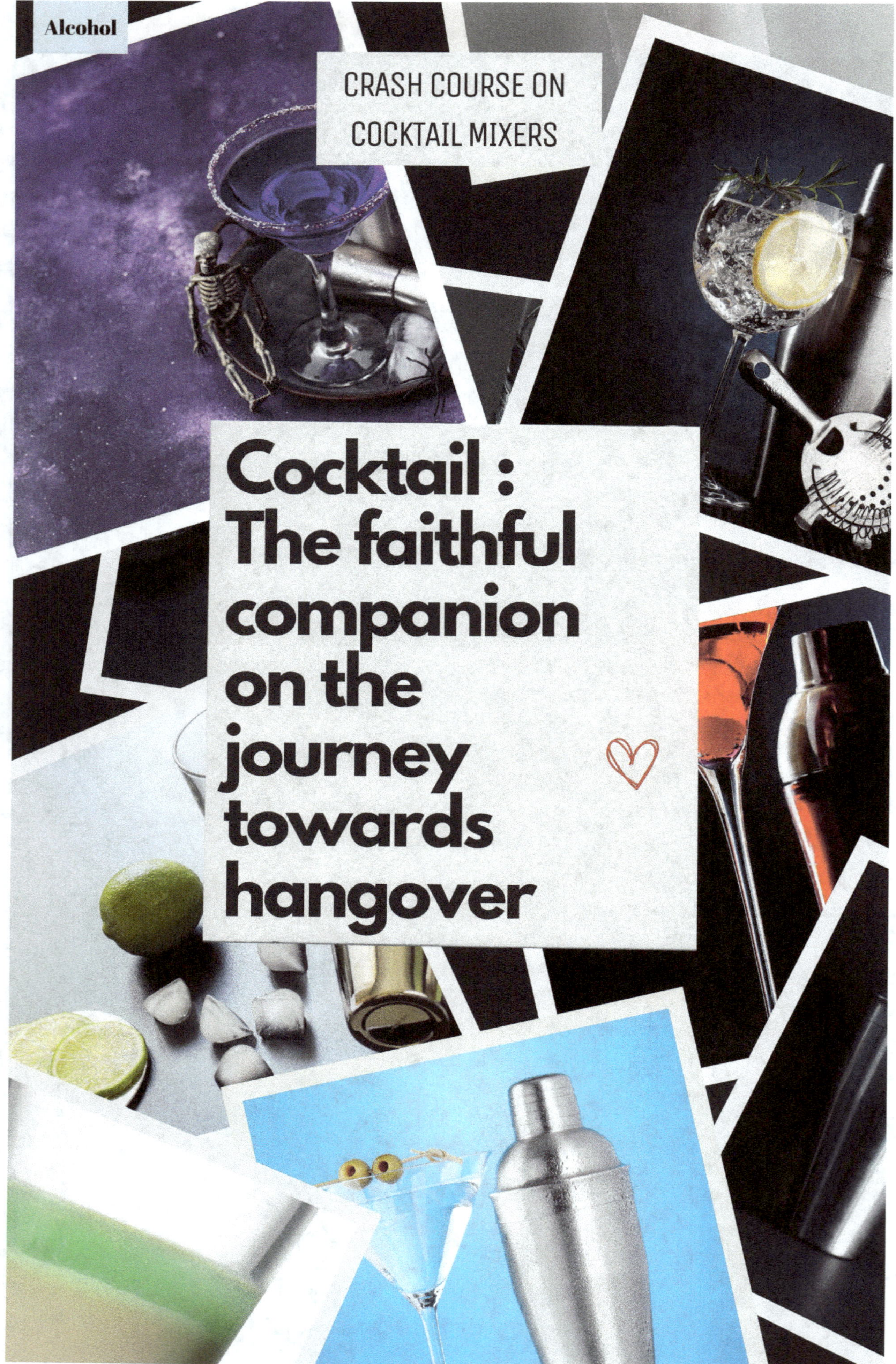

Cocktail : The faithful companion on the journey towards hangover

Grenadine

- **Country of Origin:** France
- **Primary Ingredient:** Pomegranate juice and sugar syrup
- **Taste Characteristics:** Sweet and slightly tart with a fruity flavor
- **Interesting Facts:** Grenadine is often used to add color and sweetness to cocktails. Despite its name, many commercial grenadine syrups do not contain actual pomegranate juice and are artificially flavored and colored.

Triple Sec

- **Country of Origin:** France
- **Primary Ingredient:** Orange peels
- **Taste Characteristics:** Sweet and citrusy with a strong orange flavor
- **Interesting Facts:** Triple Sec is a type of orange liqueur used in a wide range of cocktails, including the Margarita and Cosmopolitan. "Triple Sec" means "triple distilled," referring to its production process.

Angostura Bitters

- **Country of Origin:** Trinidad and Tobago
- **Primary Ingredient:** A secret blend of herbs and spices
- **Taste Characteristics:** Extremely bitter with complex herbal and spice undertones
- **Interesting Facts:** Angostura Bitters were originally developed as a medicinal tonic by a German doctor in the early 19th century. Today, they are a key ingredient in classic cocktails like the Old Fashioned and Manhattan.

Campari

- **Country of Origin:** Italy
- **Primary Ingredient:** Bitter herbs, aromatic plants, and fruit
- **Taste Characteristics:** Bitter and herbal with a hint of citrus and spice
- **Interesting Facts:** Campari is known for its distinctive red color and is a key component in cocktails like the Negroni and Americano. It has a long history dating back to the 1860s.

Coconut Cream

- **Country of Origin:** Various tropical regions
- **Primary Ingredient:** Extracted from coconut meat and combined with sugar
- **Taste Characteristics:** Sweet and creamy with a pronounced coconut flavor
- **Interesting Facts:** Coconut cream is commonly used in tropical cocktails like the Piña Colada. It adds a rich and tropical essence to drinks.

Orgeat Syrup

- **Country of Origin:** France
- **Primary Ingredient:** Almonds and sugar with a hint of orange flower water
- **Taste Characteristics:** Sweet, nutty, and with a subtle floral note
- **Interesting Facts:** Orgeat syrup is a key ingredient in tiki cocktails like the Mai Tai. It's made from almonds and has a unique flavor that adds depth and complexity to drinks.

Irish Cream Liqueur

- **Country of Origin:** Ireland
- **Primary Ingredient:** Irish whiskey, cream, and sweeteners
- **Taste Characteristics:** Sweet, creamy, and rich with a subtle whiskey flavor
- **Interesting Facts:** Baileys Irish Cream is one of the most popular brands of Irish cream liqueur. It's often enjoyed on its own over ice or used in coffee-based cocktails.

Hollywood Lines to Keep in the Back of Your Mind

Pop Culture

"Life is like a box of chocolates; you never know what you're gonna get."

Movie: "Forrest Gump" (1994)
Background: This iconic line is delivered by Forrest Gump (Tom Hanks) in the movie "Forrest Gump" (1994). The scene takes place in Savannah, Georgia, where Forrest sits on a park bench while waiting for a bus. He narrates his life story to strangers who sit next to him, recounting various events and adventures that shaped his life. This quote captures the essence of Forrest's simple yet profound outlook on life, emphasizing the unpredictability of experiences and opportunities.

"You can't handle the truth!"

Movie: "A Few Good Men" (1992)
Background: In "A Few Good Men" (1992), this quote is shouted by Colonel Nathan R. Jessup (Jack Nicholson) during a dramatic courtroom confrontation. Lieutenant Daniel Kaffee (Tom Cruise) is cross-examining Jessup about a hazing incident that led to the death of a Marine. Jessup angrily challenges Kaffee, asserting that the courtroom cannot handle the harsh realities of military life and the sacrifices made by soldiers.

"I feel the need... the need for speed."

Movie: "Top Gun" (1986, but influential in the '90s)
Background: Maverick (played by Tom Cruise) and Goose (played by Anthony Edwards) are fighter jet pilots in the United States Navy's elite Top Gun Naval Fighter Weapons School. This quote is often used as they prepare for high-speed aerial maneuvers in their F-14 Tomcat jets.

"Show me the money!"

Movie: "Jerry Maguire" (1996)
Background: Jerry Maguire (played by Tom Cruise) is a sports agent who's trying to win back the loyalty of his client, Rod Tidwell (played by Cuba Gooding Jr.). In this scene, Rod demands that Jerry prove his dedication by securing him a lucrative contract. "Show me the money!" becomes Rod's catchphrase throughout the movie.

"I'll be back."

Movie: "Terminator 2: Judgment Day" (1991)
Background: The Terminator (played by Arnold Schwarzenegger) delivers this line before leaving a police station, and it becomes one of his iconic catchphrases throughout the "Terminator" series. In the film, the Terminator promises to return while embarking on his mission to protect John Connor from a shape-shifting assassin.

"Hasta la vista, baby."

Movie: "Terminator 2: Judgment Day" (1991)
Background: The Terminator (Arnold Schwarzenegger) delivers this line with a touch of humor before dispatching an adversary with his shotgun. It adds a memorable and slightly ironic tone to his otherwise stoic character.

"You had me at 'hello.'"

Movie: "Jerry Maguire" (1996)
Background: In this romantic moment, Dorothy Boyd (played by Renée Zellweger) watches Jerry Maguire's heartfelt and desperate speech about his feelings for her. She tearfully responds with this line, conveying that she was won over from the moment he began speaking.

"You're gonna need a bigger boat."

Movie: Jaws (1975)
Background: Chief Brody (Roy Scheider) says this when he first catches sight of the enormous great white shark. It's a humorous and iconic line that underscores the danger they face. The film revolves around the hunt for a man-eating shark terrorizing a coastal town. "Jaws" is a landmark thriller directed by Steven Spielberg.

"Houston, we have a problem."

Movie: Apollo 13 (1995)
Background: This line is based on a real-life communication between the Apollo 13 spacecraft and NASA's mission control during a critical technical failure in space. It's a pivotal moment in the film as it marks the start of a life-threatening crisis for the astronauts. "Apollo 13" is a gripping and fact-based drama about the ill-fated Apollo 13 mission to the moon.

"Keep your friends close, but your enemies closer."

Movie: The Godfather Part II (1974)
Background: Michael Corleone (Al Pacino) offers this piece of advice about dealing with adversaries. He emphasizes the importance of understanding and monitoring one's enemies closely. The film is a sequel to "The Godfather" and explores the rise of Michael Corleone as a mafia leader, juxtaposed with flashbacks to the early life of his father, Vito Corleone.

"May the Force be with you."

Movie: Star Wars (1977)
Background: It is a common phrase used throughout the "Star Wars" franchise. It's an expression of goodwill and encouragement. The Force is a mystical energy that plays a central role in the series, and this phrase reflects the importance of the Force in the characters' lives. "Star Wars" is a legendary space opera franchise created by George Lucas, set in a galaxy far, far away, featuring epic battles between the forces of good (the Jedi) and evil (the Sith).

"Here's looking at you, kid."

Movie: Casablanca (1942)
Background: In "Casablanca," the quote is spoken by Rick Blaine (Humphrey Bogart) to Ilsa Lund (Ingrid Bergman). The film is set in the Moroccan city of Casablanca during World War II. Rick and Ilsa have a complicated history, and Rick uses this line as a parting phrase to Ilsa. It's a moment filled with longing and nostalgia. "Casablanca" is a classic romantic drama that explores themes of love, sacrifice, and moral choices against the backdrop of wartime intrigue.

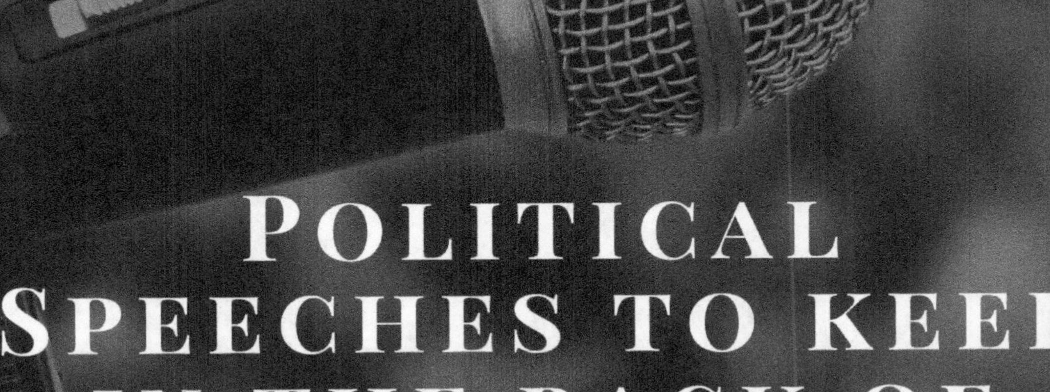

Political Speeches to keep in the back of your mind

Motivation

"I have a dream that my four little children will one day live in a nation where they will not be judged by the color of their skin but by the content of their character."
- Martin Luther King Jr.

Reference: This quote is from Martin Luther King Jr.'s iconic "I Have a Dream" speech, delivered during the March on Washington for Jobs and Freedom on August 28, 1963. It is a powerful call for racial equality and civil rights.

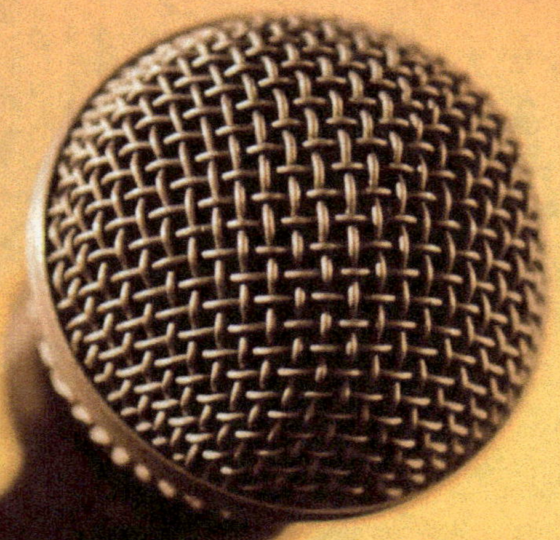

"Ask not what your country can do for you; ask what you can do for your country." - John F. Kennedy

Reference: President John F. Kennedy delivered this famous line in his inaugural address on January 20, 1961. It emphasizes civic responsibility and the idea that citizens should actively contribute to their nation's well-being.

"Tear down this wall!" - Ronald Reagan

Reference: President Ronald Reagan delivered this line in his speech at the Brandenburg Gate in Berlin on June 12, 1987, addressing the Soviet leader Mikhail Gorbachev and calling for the dismantling of the Berlin Wall, which ultimately fell in 1989, leading to the reunification of Germany.

"The only thing we have to fear is fear itself." - Franklin D. Roosevelt

Reference: President Franklin D. Roosevelt spoke these words during his first inaugural address on March 4, 1933, as the United States faced the challenges of the Great Depression. It reassured the nation in a time of crisis.

"In this world of ours in other lands, there are some people who, in times of war, must live in constant fear and hunger. That's a crime against humanity." - Eleanor Roosevelt

Reference: This quote is from a speech by Eleanor Roosevelt, the former First Lady and human rights advocate. She delivered this address in 1948 as she played a key role in drafting the Universal Declaration of Human Rights.

"We shall fight on the beaches, we shall fight on the landing grounds, we shall fight in the fields and in the streets, we shall fight in the hills; we shall never surrender." - Winston Churchill

Reference: Prime Minister Winston Churchill delivered this speech on June 4, 1940, during World War II, rallying the British people against the threat of Nazi invasion. It is a stirring call for perseverance and defiance.

"Ich bin ein Berliner." - John F. Kennedy

Reference: President John F. Kennedy uttered these words in a speech delivered in West Berlin on June 26, 1963, expressing solidarity with the people of Berlin during the Cold War. It translates to "I am a Berliner" in German.

"Mr. Gorbachev, tear down this wall!" - Ronald Reagan

Reference: President Ronald Reagan repeated a similar line to the one mentioned earlier in a speech at the Berlin Wall on June 12, 1987, urging the Soviet leader Mikhail Gorbachev to dismantle the wall separating East and West Berlin.

"Change is the law of life. And those who look only to the past or present are certain to miss the future." - John F. Kennedy

Reference: President John F. Kennedy delivered these words during a speech at the dedication of the Robert Frost Library on October 26, 1963. It underscores the importance of adaptability and progress.

Crash Course on Pull and Push Workout Routine

Why to consider a Push / Pull Based Workout Regime

Balanced Muscle Development: Push exercises primarily target the chest, shoulders, and triceps, while pull exercises focus on the back, biceps, and rear deltoids. By including both push and pull movements in your routine, you ensure balanced development of these muscle groups, reducing the risk of muscular imbalances and postural issues.

Improved Functional Strength: Pushing and pulling movements are fundamental to many daily activities and sports. A balanced push and pull workout enhances your functional strength, making everyday tasks easier and improving your performance in sports and recreational activities.

Enhanced Posture: Strengthening both the push and pull muscle groups helps maintain good posture by keeping the shoulders back and the chest open. This can alleviate common posture-related problems like rounded shoulders and forward head posture.

Injury Prevention: A balanced routine can reduce the risk of injuries by strengthening the muscles that support your joints. Stronger muscles and tendons provide better stability and support, which can help prevent strains and injuries during workouts and daily life.

Muscle Symmetry: A push and pull workout can help create balanced muscle symmetry, giving your physique an aesthetically pleasing and proportionate appearance.

Versatility: Push and pull exercises can be performed using various equipment, such as barbells, dumbbells, resistance bands, bodyweight, or gym machines. This versatility allows you to adapt your workouts to different environments and equipment availability.

Efficiency: Push and pull workouts often involve compound exercises that engage multiple muscle groups simultaneously. This efficiency allows you to work on multiple muscle groups in a single session, saving time while still delivering effective results.

Variety and Interest: The diversity of push and pull exercises keeps workouts interesting and prevents boredom. This variety can help maintain motivation and adherence to your fitness routine.

Cardiovascular Benefits: While primarily a strength-training approach, push and pull workouts can also provide cardiovascular benefits when performed with minimal rest between sets. This can help improve endurance and overall cardiovascular fitness.

Understand the Push and Pull Movements

Push Movements: These exercises involve extending or pushing a weight or your body away from you. They primarily target the muscles responsible for these movements, such as the chest (pectoralis major), shoulders (anterior deltoids), and triceps.

Pull Movements: These exercises involve contracting or pulling a weight or your body toward you. They target muscles involved in pulling actions, including the back (latissimus dorsi), biceps, and rear deltoids.

Select Appropriate Exercises

Exercise selection should align with your fitness goals and skill level.

If you're a beginner, start with basic exercises like push-ups, bodyweight rows, and dumbbell curls to build a foundation of strength and technique.
As you progress, incorporate more advanced exercises like bench presses, pull-ups, barbell rows, and compound movements that engage multiple muscle groups.
Customizing your exercise selection to suit your goals ensures efficient and effective progress.

Design Your Workout

You can organize your workout into distinct push and pull days or incorporate both types of movements into each session.

For example, a push day might include exercises like bench presses, overhead presses, push-ups, and tricep dips, while a pull day might consist of pull-ups, bent-over rows, bicep curls, and face pulls.

Alternately, you can use full-body workouts that include both push and pull exercises if you prefer more frequent workouts.

The number of repetitions (reps) and sets you perform will depend on your specific goals.
For strength training, use lower reps (3-5 reps per set) with heavier weights to maximize strength gains.
If hypertrophy (muscle growth) is your aim, opt for moderate reps (8-12 reps per set) with weights that challenge your muscles.
Endurance-focused workouts can involve higher reps (15-20 reps per set) with lighter weights.

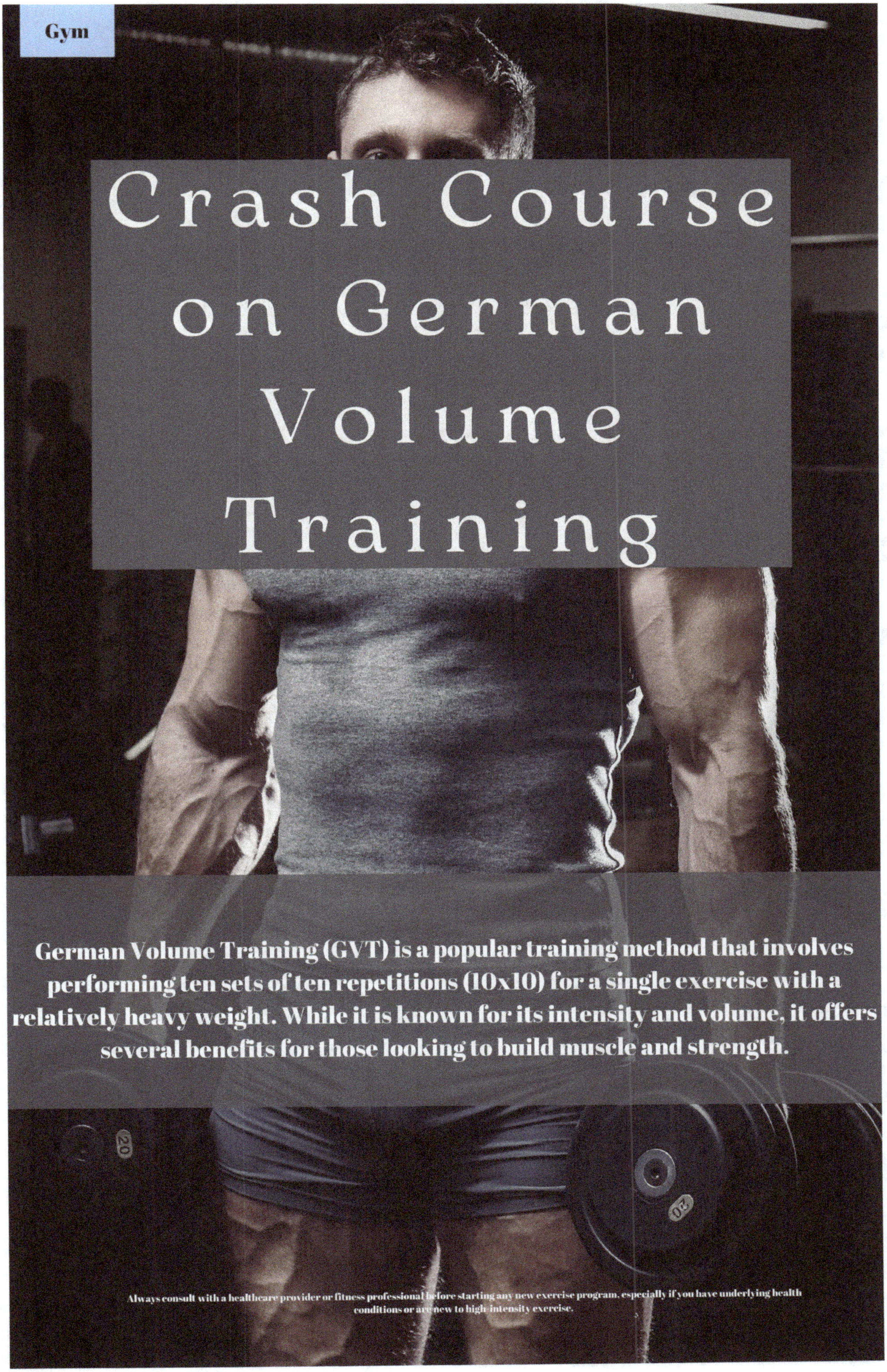

Crash Course on German Volume Training

German Volume Training (GVT) is a popular training method that involves performing ten sets of ten repetitions (10x10) for a single exercise with a relatively heavy weight. While it is known for its intensity and volume, it offers several benefits for those looking to build muscle and strength.

Always consult with a healthcare provider or fitness professional before starting any new exercise program, especially if you have underlying health conditions or are new to high-intensity exercise.

Advantages of German Volume Training

Muscle Hypertrophy: GVT is highly effective for stimulating muscle growth. The high volume and time under tension (TUT) created by performing ten sets of ten reps can lead to muscle hypertrophy, making it a popular choice among bodybuilders.

Strength Gains: Although GVT primarily targets muscle size, it can also lead to strength gains, especially for those who are relatively new to resistance training. The consistent practice of lifting heavy weights for multiple sets helps build strength over time.

Efficiency: GVT is time-efficient because it focuses on a single exercise for a large portion of the workout. This can be beneficial for individuals with busy schedules who want to maximize their training effectiveness in a shorter time frame.

Increased Work Capacity: Performing ten sets of ten reps challenges your work capacity and endurance. Over time, this can improve your ability to handle more volume and intensity, which can benefit other training programs.
Mental Toughness: GVT can be mentally demanding due to the high volume and repetition scheme. It can help improve mental toughness, discipline, and focus, which can translate to better performance in other aspects of life and training.

Variation and Plateau Breaking: If you've hit a plateau in your training, GVT can be an effective way to shock your muscles and break through stagnation. The high volume and intensity can stimulate new muscle growth.

Structural Balance: GVT typically involves compound exercises, which promote structural balance by targeting multiple muscle groups. This can help prevent imbalances and reduce the risk of injury.

Minimal Equipment: GVT workouts often require minimal equipment, making it accessible to individuals who have limited access to a gym or prefer training at home.

Customizable: While the traditional GVT program involves ten sets of ten reps, you can modify the intensity, exercise selection, and rest intervals to tailor the program to your specific goals and fitness level.

Recovery Focus: GVT emphasizes proper recovery between sets, which can teach the importance of rest and recuperation in a training program. This can help prevent overtraining and injury.

Metabolic Stress: The high volume and short rest periods in GVT can create metabolic stress, which may contribute to increased calorie burn and fat loss, making it a useful tool for individuals aiming to reduce body fat.

Crash Course on HIIT

High-Intensity Interval Training (HIIT) is a popular and effective workout strategy that involves short bursts of intense exercise followed by brief periods of rest or lower-intensity activity. HIIT offers numerous benefits and can be an efficient way to improve cardiovascular fitness, burn calories, and build endurance.

Always consult with a healthcare provider or fitness professional before starting any new exercise program, especially if you have underlying health conditions or are new to high-intensity exercise.

Advantages of HIIT

Time Efficiency: HIIT workouts are typically shorter than traditional steady-state cardio workouts because they are so intense. You can get a highly effective workout in as little as 20-30 minutes.

Increased Calorie Burn: HIIT elevates your heart rate and metabolism, resulting in a significant calorie burn during and after the workout. This is known as the "afterburn" effect or excess post-exercise oxygen consumption (EPOC).

Improved Cardiovascular Fitness: HIIT can improve your aerobic and anaerobic capacity, enhancing your heart and lung function. It can also help reduce your risk of heart disease and improve overall cardiovascular health.

Fat Loss: HIIT has been shown to be effective at reducing body fat percentage, especially when combined with a balanced diet. The combination of increased calorie burn and muscle engagement contributes to fat loss.

Preservation of Muscle Mass: Unlike steady-state cardio, which may lead to muscle loss over time, HIIT can help preserve lean muscle mass while promoting fat loss. This is especially beneficial for individuals looking to maintain or build muscle.

Variety and Versatility: HIIT workouts can be adapted to various activities, including running, cycling, swimming, bodyweight exercises, and even strength training. This versatility makes it suitable for individuals with different preferences and fitness levels.

Metabolic Benefits: HIIT can improve insulin sensitivity and glucose regulation, potentially reducing the risk of type 2 diabetes.

Time and Location Flexibility: You can perform HIIT workouts virtually anywhere, making them convenient for individuals with busy schedules or limited access to a gym.

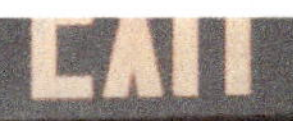

To define a workout based on the principles of HIIT, follow these steps:

Choose Your Exercise: Select an exercise or a combination of exercises that can be performed at high intensity. Common choices include sprints, cycling, jumping jacks, burpees, kettlebell swings, and bodyweight exercises like squats, push-ups, and mountain climbers.

Warm-Up: Begin with a 5-10 minute warm-up that includes light cardio or dynamic stretching to prepare your muscles and joints.

Interval Structure: Determine the work and rest intervals. HIIT typically involves 20-60 seconds of intense effort followed by 10-60 seconds of rest or low-intensity recovery. The work-to-rest ratio can vary based on your fitness level and goals.

Set the Number of Rounds: Decide how many rounds or cycles you will complete. Beginners might start with 3-4 rounds, while more advanced individuals can aim for 5-8 rounds or more.

Execute the Workout: Perform the high-intensity intervals with maximal effort during the work periods, followed by active recovery or rest during the rest periods. Maintain proper form throughout.

Cool Down: Finish the workout with a 5-10 minute cooldown that includes static stretching to promote flexibility and aid in recovery.

Progressive Overload: As you become fitter, gradually increase the intensity by reducing rest intervals, increasing work intervals, or incorporating more challenging exercises.

Frequency: You can include HIIT workouts in your routine 2-4 times per week, depending on your goals and recovery capacity. Allow at least 48 hours between intense HIIT sessions to ensure proper recovery.

Crash Course on Protein Powder

High-Intensity Interval Training (HIIT) is a popular and effective workout strategy that involves short bursts of intense exercise followed by brief periods of rest or lower-intensity activity. HIIT offers numerous benefits and can be an efficient way to improve cardiovascular fitness, burn calories, and build endurance.

Before starting any supplement regimen, including creatine, it's advisable to consult with a healthcare professional or a registered dietitian, especially if you have underlying health conditions or are taking medication.

WHEY PROTEIN

Protein Source: Whey protein is derived from milk during the cheese-making process and is considered a complete protein, containing all essential amino acids.

Protein-to-Carbs Ratio: Whey protein isolate typically has a higher protein content with very low carbs (often less than 1 gram of carbohydrates per serving). Whey protein concentrate may have slightly more carbs (around 3-4 grams per serving).

Recommended Timing: Whey protein is rapidly absorbed, making it an excellent choice for post-workout recovery. Consuming whey protein within 30 minutes to 2 hours after exercise can help maximize muscle protein synthesis and recovery.

Protein Source: Like whey, casein is derived from milk but is digested more slowly. It's also a complete protein.

Protein-to-Carbs Ratio: Casein protein powders typically have a low carbohydrate content, similar to whey protein isolates.

Recommended Timing: Due to its slow digestion, casein protein is often consumed before bedtime to provide a sustained release of amino acids during sleep, helping with muscle repair and recovery.

CASEIN PROTEIN

Before starting any supplement regimen, including creatine, it's advisable to consult with a healthcare professional.

PEA PROTEIN

Protein Source: Pea protein is plant-based and derived from yellow split peas. It's suitable for vegetarians and vegans.

Protein-to-Carbs Ratio: Pea protein powders generally have a favorable protein-to-carbs ratio, with minimal carbohydrates.

Recommended Timing: Pea protein can be consumed at various times throughout the day, similar to whey protein. It's versatile and can be used for pre- or post-workout shakes or as a protein source in meals or snacks.

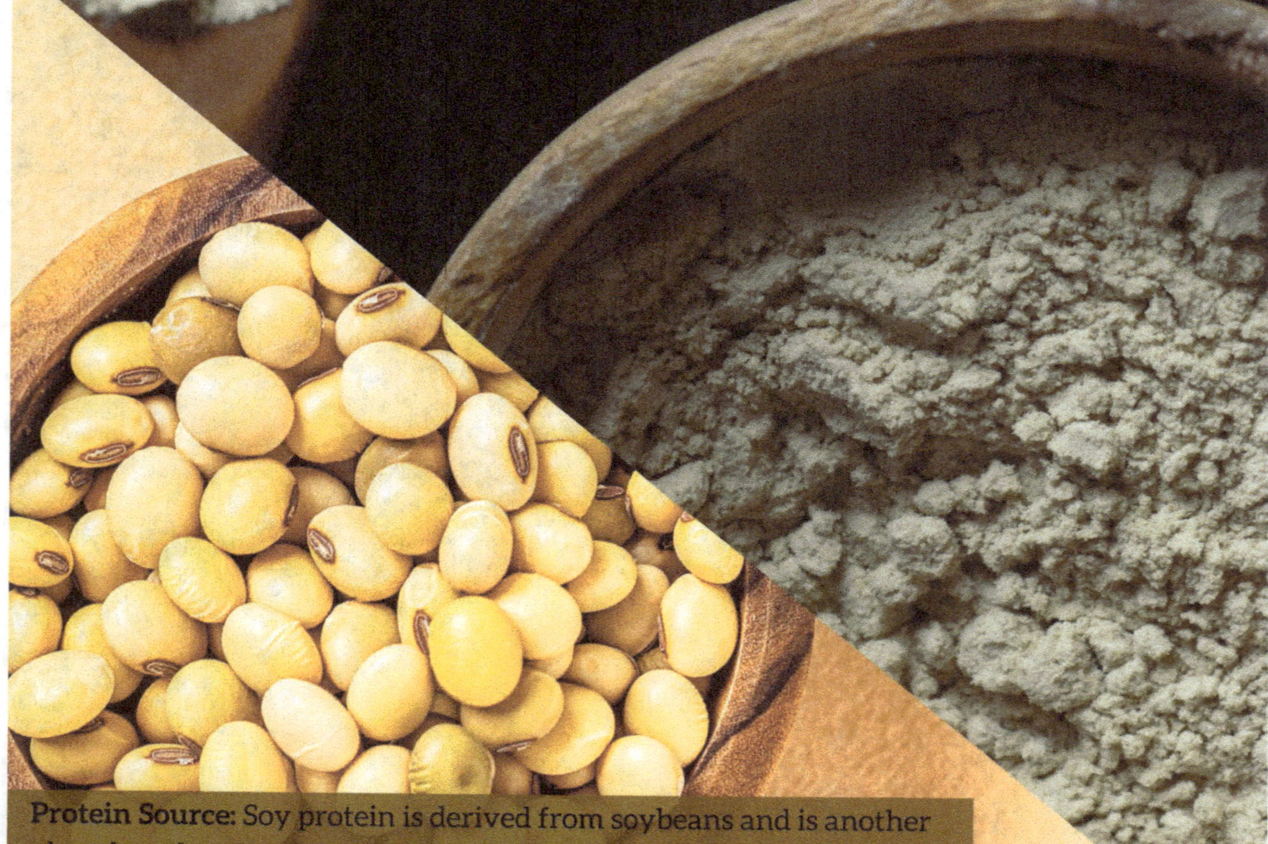

Protein Source: Soy protein is derived from soybeans and is another plant-based option that contains all essential amino acids.

Protein-to-Carbs Ratio: Soy protein powders typically have a low carbohydrate content, similar to whey and pea proteins.

Recommended Timing: Soy protein can be consumed at various times, including pre- or post-workout. Some people also use it as a meal replacement.

SOY PROTEIN

Crash Course on Creatine

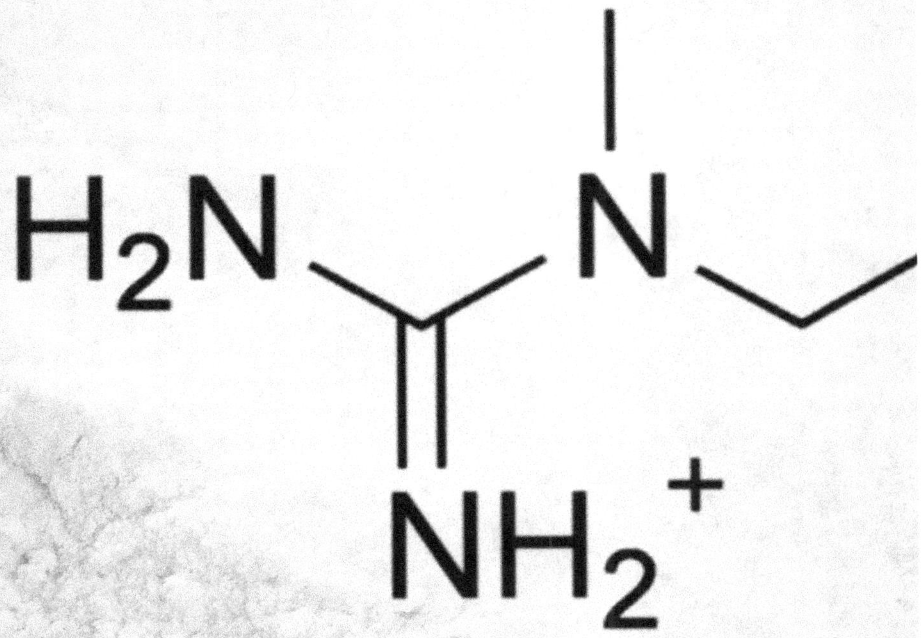

Creatine is a naturally occurring compound found in small amounts in certain foods and synthesized by the body. It's one of the most extensively studied and popular supplements among athletes and fitness enthusiasts. It is primarily known for its potential benefits in enhancing performance, particularly in activities that involve short bursts of high-intensity effort.

Benefits of Creatine

Improved Exercise Performance: Creatine has been shown to enhance high-intensity, short-duration activities, such as weightlifting, sprinting, and high-intensity interval training (HIIT). It helps increase the availability of energy during these activities, which can lead to improved strength, power, and performance.

Increased Muscle Mass: Creatine may promote muscle growth by increasing water content in muscle cells and stimulating protein synthesis. This can lead to greater muscle volume and hypertrophy over time.

Enhanced Muscle Recovery: Some studies suggest that creatine supplementation can reduce muscle damage and inflammation, potentially aiding in faster recovery between intense workouts.

Brain Health: Emerging research suggests that creatine may have cognitive benefits, such as improved memory and brain function. It may be particularly useful in situations where cognitive function is compromised, such as during sleep deprivation or under high-stress conditions.

Potential Medical Benefits: Creatine supplementation is being explored for its potential therapeutic uses in certain medical conditions, including neuromuscular diseases and neurodegenerative disorders.

Before starting any supplement regimen, including creatine, it's advisable to consult with a healthcare professional or a registered dietitian, especially if you have underlying health conditions or are taking medication.

Risks of Creatine

Digestive Issues: Some individuals may experience gastrointestinal discomfort when taking creatine, such as bloating, cramping, or diarrhea. Staying hydrated and spreading the dose throughout the day can help minimize these side effects.

Weight Gain: Creatine can lead to an initial increase in body weight, primarily due to water retention within muscle cells. This is not the same as fat gain and typically levels out over time.

Kidney Strain: There is no conclusive evidence to suggest that creatine supplementation is harmful to healthy kidneys when used within recommended dosages. However, individuals with preexisting kidney issues should consult a healthcare professional before using creatine.

Dehydration: Creatine may increase water retention in muscles, potentially leading to dehydration if an individual does not consume enough fluids. It's essential to stay adequately hydrated while using creatine.

Recommended Timing for Creatine Supplementation

The timing of creatine supplementation can vary depending on individual preferences and goals. Here are a few common approaches:

- **Loading Phase:** Some people choose to begin creatine supplementation with a loading phase, which involves taking a higher dose (around 20 grams) divided into smaller servings throughout the day for 5-7 days. After this period, they switch to a maintenance dose.

- **Maintenance Phase:** Once the loading phase is completed, a maintenance dose of 3-5 grams per day is typically sufficient to maintain elevated creatine levels in the muscles.

- **Timing Around Workouts:** Many individuals take creatine either before or after their workouts. This timing can help maximize its potential benefits for exercise performance and muscle recovery.

- **Consistent Daily Dosing:** Some people prefer to take creatine at the same time every day, regardless of their workout schedule. This approach ensures a steady supply of creatine in the body.

Before starting any supplement regimen, including creatine, it's advisable to consult with a healthcare professional or a registered dietitian, especially if you have underlying health conditions or are taking medication.

Crash Course on Additional Gym Supplements

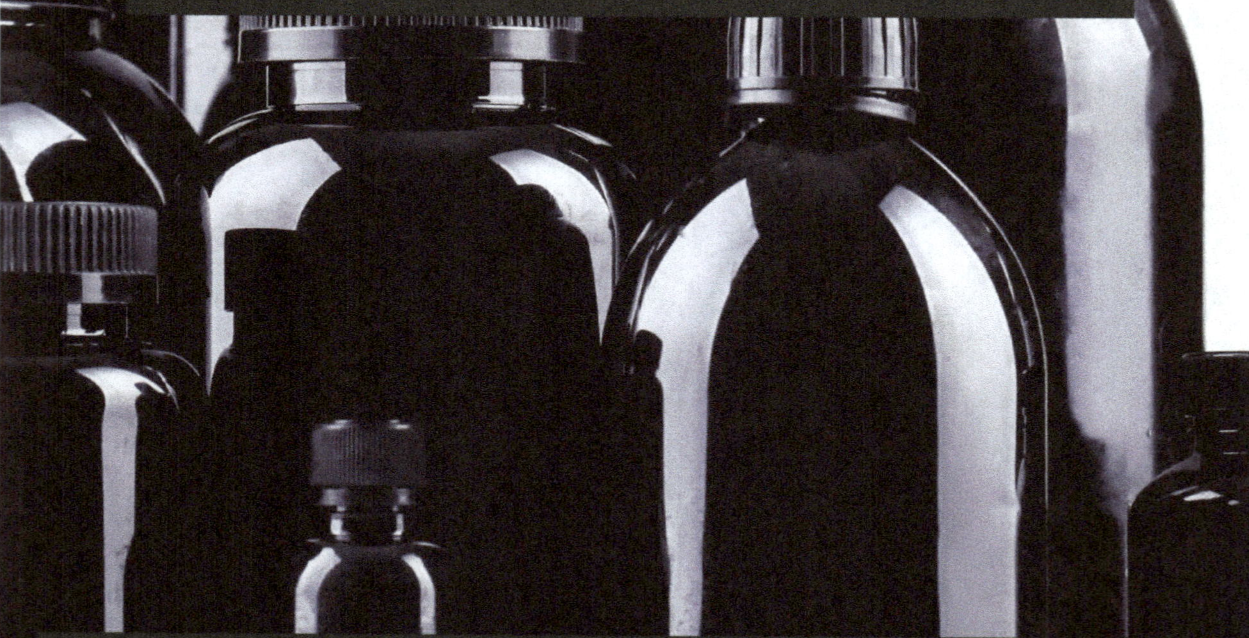

Creatine is a naturally occurring compound found in small amounts in certain foods and synthesized by the body. It's one of the most extensively studied and popular supplements among athletes and fitness enthusiasts. It is primarily known for its potential benefits in enhancing performance, particularly in activities that involve short bursts of high-intensity effort.

It's important to note that while supplements can be beneficial for some individuals, they should not replace a balanced and nutrient-dense diet. Prior to starting any supplement regimen, consult with a healthcare provider or a registered dietitian to ensure they are safe and appropriate for your specific needs and goals. Additionally, follow the recommended dosages and guidelines provided by the manufacturer and consider the potential risks associated with each supplement.

Branched-Chain Amino Acids (BCAAs)

Benefits: BCAAs (leucine, isoleucine, and valine) can help reduce muscle soreness, improve endurance, and support muscle protein synthesis.

Risks: When used as a supplement, side effects are rare. However, they should not be a sole source of dietary protein.

Recommended Timing: BCAAs can be taken before, during, or after workouts to help reduce muscle fatigue and promote recovery.

Pre-Workout Supplements

Benefits: Pre-workout supplements typically contain caffeine, amino acids, and other ingredients that may increase energy, focus, and exercise performance.

Risks: Some individuals may be sensitive to the caffeine content and experience jitters, increased heart rate, or sleep disturbances.

Recommended Timing: Take pre-workout supplements 20-30 minutes before exercise to maximize their effects.

Beta-Alanine

Benefits: Beta-alanine can enhance muscular endurance by increasing intramuscular carnosine levels, which help buffer acid build-up during high-intensity exercise.

Risks: The most common side effect is a harmless tingling sensation (paresthesia). It's generally considered safe when used within recommended dosages.

Recommended Timing: Beta-alanine can be taken as a daily supplement, and timing doesn't have to be precise. Consistency in daily dosing is essential to build up carnosine levels over time.

It's important to note that while supplements can be beneficial for some individuals, they should not replace a balanced and nutrient-dense diet. Prior to starting any supplement regimen, consult with a healthcare provider or a registered dietitian to ensure they are safe and appropriate for your specific needs and goals. Additionally, follow the recommended dosages and guidelines provided by the manufacturer and consider the potential risks associated with each supplement.

Nitric Oxide Boosters (e.g., L-arginine)

Benefits: These supplements may enhance blood flow, muscle pump, and oxygen delivery to muscles during workouts.

Risks: Some individuals may experience gastrointestinal discomfort. Their effectiveness can vary among individuals.

Recommended Timing: Take nitric oxide boosters 30-60 minutes before workouts to maximize their effects.

Post-Workout Carbohydrates

Benefits: Consuming carbohydrates after exercise helps replenish glycogen stores and support recovery. Combining carbs with protein can further enhance muscle repair.

Risks: Excessive carbohydrate intake may lead to unwanted weight gain if not matched with energy expenditure.

Recommended Timing: Consume post-workout carbohydrates and protein within 30 minutes to 2 hours after exercise to optimize recovery.

It's important to note that while supplements can be beneficial for some individuals, they should not replace a balanced and nutrient-dense diet. Prior to starting any supplement regimen, consult with a healthcare provider or a registered dietitian to ensure they are safe and appropriate for your specific needs and goals. Additionally, follow the recommended dosages and guidelines provided by the manufacturer and consider the potential risks associated with each supplement.

First lessons are the most important ones

Chances are you've known how to make yourself ejaculate since you first discovered masturbation as a teenager. Well treat that as an experience of offense; add a girl in the mix and you now need to learn how to defend.

And the best way to defend is to understand the lay of the ground. One can do this by taking the first few sexual encounters more as a lesson in sex, rather than a jaunty roll in the sack.

The payoff of putting her pleasure first, will let you understand what works for you the best and also learn directly from the horses mouth on how to actually win the race. Now this is true, that the experience itself might be sullied for you, but it will make it all worth in the long run especially when you will always have return calls.

BASICS OF EATING DESSERT

Meaningful Education

WALK BEFORE YOU RUN

Step 1 : Pre heating the Dessert

Start off with kissing her mouth down to her breasts. Keep kissing her body as you lower yourself to her waist and hips. As you get closer to her panties, place a hand between her legs and slowly spread them apart. During your journey down, make note of any special spots that especially create arousal and jot them down in your memory for later or future use. These are known as erogenous zones and some of them might surprise you.

Step 2 : Handling the Packaging

Panties can actually add more fun to the whole mix so don't worry about taking them off just yet. Instead, kiss her vagina through her panties and even squeeze it ever so lightly with your lips. Running your tongue over the panty from her vagina to her clit might be exciting too.

Step 3 : Patience patience patience

Now try to take your mind (and senses) of the nether regions and move southwards towards her knees. Continue the flow of kisses along her inner thigh applying little pleasure. Move down one leg and up the other. Make as far down as the knee, further down might not bring the same level of results. **Pro tip :** If she likes it a bit rougher, then you can safely leave a hickey between her legs and it can be your little secret.

Step 4 : Unwrap

If so far she has played sport and hasn't herself taken her panty's off then it's your job to do the honours. Be soft and sensual about it, keeping in mind with the moment.

Step 5 : Ahem

Start off with slowly kissing and licking (ever so softly) all around her vagina and clit. Make sure that your lips are making only a tiny amount of contact with her vagina and clit; objective here is tease and excite her and build the anticipation for the acts to come

Step 6 : Bon appetite

Depending on your skill level you can now go the beginner or expert way of eating your dessert

Beginner : Rolling Stones knew how to Rock n Roll

Start by taking your tongue out and hang all the way to your chin, make it wide and flat and relax it.

Make sure that it is completely covered with saliva, and bring it her vagina, moving it from the bottom of her vagina all the way to the top, so that it slowly passes next to her clit. Point to note is that your tongue isn't making the moves, but your head is. As the head moves, the tongue follows.

Keep repeating the motion till she cums.

Now you will ask, is that it?
Well.. no! These are the basics, now comes the part where you have to keep your senses on to read how her body is reacting to your motions.

If your motions aren't hearing, feeling or seeing any major reaction from her like clutching your hair or linen, bodily tensions signalling an orgasm, etc. then try increasing the speed of your head motions or apply additional pressure from your tongue making more deliberate passes on the clit.

One tip that can help is to communicate, ask her what is working for her and if you can change any of the metric at play from your side (speed, pressure, breath).

Pro Tips for the Beginner Method :

Steady Pace : Most women appreciate a steady pace of this beginner method, however maintaining the same isn't the easiest and will require significant practice.

Edging : This is possible when you are well versed with your partner's body. It requires to know when she is about to cum, and for you to then slow down your motions thereby delaying her orgasm. Which when it eventually comes, is significantly more intensified.

Expert : You suck

Start by making an 'O' with your mouth and cover your lips with saliva.
Gently put his O on her clit and start sucking, thereby slowly bringing her clit into the warmth of your mouth.

From here on you can do try one or a mixture of the below and adapt as you feel her body react to your actions.

Constant – Probably the easiest way is by keeping a constant level of suction. For some women, this will be all you need to help them reach climax.
Rhythmic – Performing this will mean that you will be sucking and releasing the pressure rhythmically, pulling her clit in and out of your mouth and releasing it. This can also be done while listening to the rhythms of a song you are playing in the background..
Hard, then slow release – You will need to suddenly apply a strong level of suction to her clit, before releasing it slowly. Rinse & repeat.
Licking – When you suck her clit into your mouth, try holding it there, and you use your tongue to massage her clit. As mentioned earlier, vary the speed and pressure while figuring out what she enjoys most. **Pro tip :** Some girls like it if you write the letter 'S' on her clit with your tongue while doing the 'O'

ADVANCED LESSONS IN BAKING DESSERT

Master Degree

RUN BEFORE YOU FLY

Additional tips and tricks of the trade

Giving Her The Finger

Using your fingers when you are eating her pussy can be an amazing experience for both you and the girl. It gives you the opportunity to give her more stimulation, stimulate her simultaneously internally and externally, and provides her with lots of variation. The number of fingers depends on the girl and her comfort level. Communication is very important for such an act and is highly encouraged.

Licking Her Clit while Fingering Her G Spot

Licking her clit while you finger her G Spot is a great way to add your hands in the mix. Scientists have even found that oral and manual sex (fingering) along with deep kissing are the three activities most likely to get a woman cum.

Lick Her Clit, Finger Her G Spot & Play With Her Ass

We now enter the ass zone. Did you know that the asshole has the highest nerve endings in the whole human body? However, bringing this in the mix depends purely on the woman you are with. Some like it while others simply hate it. Therefore, communicate before you go there.

If she likes getting her salad tossed then go about licking her clit, finger massaging her G Spot, and bring your other hand in the mix and gently play around with her asshole while making no penetration. In this method the main course of dessert is still the clit, asshole is simply the garnishing on the side.

However, from here on you can go multiple ways.

You can move on to eating her ass.

Penetrating the ass with your tongue or your fingers. Keep in mind to not use the same fingers as you had used for fingering her pussy to avoid giving her any infections.

Basically, experiment! And adapt based on the comfort level of your partner.

AVOID ADDING SALT TO DESSERTS

Crash Course on Avoiding Crashes

TRICK TO ALWAYS ROLLING 6

All sexual acts must be done between consenting adults.

Don't use the alphabet

A common misconception, spread mostly through movies in the 90s is that drawing alphabets with your tongue on the clit is pleasurable. Well, it is not. If anything you might stumble on to spots which are pleasurable but you won't be spending any time on them and this method is highly inconsistent. Only exception is some cases is the 'S' while doing the 'O'.

Be consistent

Being inconsistent is a great way to frustrate your girl and make it near impossible for her to orgasm. In other words, you should aim to use the same rhythm, speed, and pressure when you go down on her, especially as she's close to cumming. Again the exception is the advanced strategy when you are trying to edge her.

Not every woman wants to get oral or even wants an orgasm

Remember each woman is special and might not be interested in receiveing oral sex or even have interest in having an orgasm. Be mindful of her choices and adapt yourself accordingly.

Food is a bad idea

Licking cream off your partner's body can be incredibly erotic and fun. But licking it off her pussy can cause serious problems. Some food particles can make their way into her vagina and cause irritation or a yeast infection or even worse. For this reason, you should avoid putting cream, chocolate sauce or any other food on or near her vagina.

Do not imitate porn

Trying to imitate porn during sex or when fingering her or when eating her pussy is usually a bad idea. Porn is filmed to look good on screen, and that's it. Porn directors don't particularly care whether or not the actors are enjoying it and as a result, porn provides a shitty way to learn good pussy eating technique.

SAY YES TO YOGA

Mastering the Basics

THE PRECURSOR TO KAMASUTRA

All sexual acts must be done between consenting adults.

Improved Flexibility and Stamina:
- Poses:
  - Downward-Facing Dog (Adho Mukha Svanasana): This pose helps stretch and strengthen the entire body, including the back, legs, and shoulders, enhancing overall flexibility.
  - Bridge Pose (Setu Bandhasana): It stretches the spine and chest and strengthens the back muscles and the pelvic floor.
- **Benefits:** Enhanced flexibility and stamina gained through yoga can make it easier to maintain various sexual positions, allowing for more enjoyable and varied experiences in the bedroom.

Stress Reduction:
- Poses:
  - **Child's Pose (Balasana):** This gentle, restorative pose can induce relaxation and alleviate stress and anxiety.
  - **Corpse Pose (Savasana):** Savasana at the end of a yoga session involves complete relaxation and can help reduce stress and promote a sense of calm.
- **Benefits:** Reducing stress through yoga can lead to improved sexual performance by reducing performance anxiety and promoting a relaxed state of mind.

Enhanced Blood Circulation:
- Pose:
  - **Legs Up the Wall Pose (Viparita Karani):** This inversion pose encourages blood flow to the pelvic region, which can help with erectile function.
- **Benefits:** Better blood circulation, especially in the genital area, can lead to stronger and longer-lasting erections, improving overall sexual performance.

Mind-Body Connection:
- Poses:
  - **Mindful Breathing:** Yoga emphasizes conscious, deep breathing techniques that encourage mindfulness and a stronger mind-body connection.
  - **Tree Pose (Vrikshasana):** This balance pose requires focus and concentration, enhancing the connection between the body and mind.
- **Benefits:** Practicing mindfulness and being attuned to sensations and responses during sexual activity can lead to increased sexual satisfaction and better performance.

Increased Relaxation:
- **Poses:**
  - **Corpse Pose (Savasana):** As mentioned earlier, Savasana is excellent for promoting deep relaxation.
  - **Seated Forward Bend (Paschimottanasana):** This pose helps release tension in the back and hamstrings, promoting relaxation.
- **Benefits:** A relaxed state of mind and body can be helpful in managing performance anxiety and creating a more fulfilling sexual experience.

Pelvic Floor Strength:
- **Pose:**
  - **Mula Bandha (Root Lock):** While not a traditional yoga pose, Mula Bandha is an internal lock involving the contraction of the pelvic floor muscles, which can be practiced during various yoga poses.
- **Benefits:** Strengthening the pelvic floor muscles can lead to better control over ejaculation and improved overall sexual performance.

Hormone Balance:
- **Poses:**
  - **Camel Pose (Ustrasana):** This backbend stimulates the thyroid gland, which can help regulate hormones.
  - **Fish Pose (Matsyasana):** It stretches the thyroid and parathyroid glands, potentially supporting hormone balance.
- **Benefits:** While yoga may help promote hormone balance indirectly through stress reduction and overall well-being, specific poses can target glands that play a role in hormone regulation.

COMMUNICATION

Mastering the Basics

THE FINE LINE BETWEEN BEING AN APE AND A MAN

Communication Builds Trust: Open and honest communication fosters trust between partners. When you both feel safe discussing your desires, boundaries, and concerns, it strengthens the emotional connection in your relationship.

Understanding Each Other's Needs: Every individual has unique sexual preferences and desires. Discussing these openly allows you to gain a deeper understanding of what each partner enjoys and finds satisfying. This knowledge can lead to more fulfilling sexual experiences.

Consent and Boundaries: Clear communication is essential for establishing consent and respecting each other's boundaries. Consent should be enthusiastic, informed, and ongoing. Discussing boundaries ensures that both partners feel safe and respected during sexual activities.

Conflict Resolution: Misunderstandings or disagreements related to sex can lead to frustration and resentment. Open communication allows you to address and resolve issues promptly, preventing them from negatively impacting your relationship.

Variety and Exploration: Sex can become routine over time, leading to boredom. Honest conversations about trying new things, fantasies, or different sexual experiences can inject excitement and variety into your sex life.

Emotional Connection: Sex is not just physical; it's deeply connected to emotions. Talking openly about your desires and experiences can create a stronger emotional bond between partners, enhancing intimacy and satisfaction.

Reducing Performance Anxiety: Many individuals experience performance anxiety, which can negatively affect sexual performance. Open communication allows you to express your feelings and concerns, reducing anxiety and helping you both relax and enjoy the moment.

Empowerment and Autonomy: Open conversations empower both partners to express themselves and make informed choices about their sexual experiences. It reinforces the idea that both partners have agency in their sexual lives.

All sexual acts must be done between consenting adults.

BREASTS

Mastering the Basics

NATURES BOUNTY AT ITS BEST

Guide to Help Navigate the Mounts and Valley of the Breast

Warm up : Do not give in to the temptation immediately, instead start of by warming the body up. Potentially starting with massaging the scalp and moving your way to the shoulders and then taking the road to the breasts with a short detour on the back.

Female body is covered with special erogenous zones and the journey to the breasts can lead you on to them quite easily. Now when at the breasts itself, try embracing, stroking, and touching the skin around the boobs in pleasurable ways like kissing, sucking, licking to make the moves pleasurable to both you and her.

Take your time : Take your time brushing gently and casually up against the sides of the breasts, and the folds beneath them so that they're aching for you to wrap your full hands right around them.

Use circular motion : Lightly massage your partner's breasts and areolas with large, circular yet gentle strokes. You can also squeeze the entire breast to increase the anticipation.

Trace a swirl from the outside in : Trace the tip of your finger from the outer edges of the breast, and slowly circle your way to the center. Remember not to rush but rather enjoy every sensation, moment, contour and texture along the way.

Increase the tempo : Rub the nipples with your fingers, slowly at first, because nerve endings in areolas make them sensitive to touch. Then gradually increase your speed and pressure as your partner becomes more aroused.

TOYS

Mastering the Basics

HAVING AN EXTRA HAND NEVER HURTS

Enhanced Stimulation: Sex toys are designed to provide unique and intense sensations that can be difficult to achieve through manual stimulation alone. They can stimulate erogenous zones more effectively, leading to heightened pleasure and orgasms.

Increased Stamina: Some sex toys, such as cock rings or penis sleeves, can help men maintain firmer erections and delay ejaculation. This extended stamina can lead to longer-lasting and more satisfying sexual encounters.

Exploration and Variety: Sex toys can introduce novelty and variety into your sexual routine. Trying different toys can prevent sexual boredom and keep the excitement alive in your relationship.

Improved Performance Confidence: For men who may have performance anxiety or concerns about their sexual abilities, incorporating sex toys can alleviate pressure. Knowing that you have additional tools to enhance pleasure can boost confidence in the bedroom.

Enhanced Partner Pleasure: Sex toys are not only for solo play; they can also be incorporated into partnered sex. Many couples find that using toys together can lead to more intense and enjoyable shared experiences. Toys can stimulate both partners simultaneously, leading to mutual satisfaction.

Learning and Communication: Exploring sex toys together encourages open communication about desires, boundaries, and preferences. This can strengthen the emotional connection between partners and lead to a deeper understanding of each other's needs.

Long-Distance Intimacy: In today's interconnected world, some sex toys are designed for long-distance couples. These toys can be controlled remotely through smartphones, allowing partners to maintain intimacy and pleasure, even when separated by distance.

PINEAPPLE JUICE

Mastering the Basics

MAKE YOURSELF TASTE BETTER

Reasons why pineapple juice is considered good for sexual life

Vitamin C Content: Pineapple juice is rich in vitamin C, which is an antioxidant. Antioxidants help protect the body's cells from oxidative stress, which can damage blood vessels and reduce blood flow. Healthy blood flow is essential for maintaining erectile function.

Bromelain: Pineapple juice contains bromelain, an enzyme with anti-inflammatory properties. Some studies suggest that bromelain may help reduce inflammation and improve blood circulation. Improved circulation can contribute to better erectile function.

Improved Taste and Smell: Pineapple juice is often mentioned as a food that can positively impact the taste and smell of bodily fluids, including semen and vaginal secretions. While the scientific evidence on this topic is limited, some people believe that consuming pineapple juice can make bodily fluids taste and smell sweeter.

Hydration: Staying well-hydrated is important for overall health and can indirectly benefit sexual performance. Dehydration can lead to fatigue and reduced stamina, which can affect sexual activity negatively. Drinking fluids, including pineapple juice, can help maintain adequate hydration levels.

Mood and Energy: Pineapple juice, like other fruits and juices, contains natural sugars that can provide a quick energy boost. Feeling energized and in a good mood can contribute to a more enjoyable sexual experience.

All sexual acts must be done between consenting adults.

CRASH COURSE ON GOLF

GOOD WALK SPOILED

-Mark Twain

A Brief History Lesson

Golf, as it is recognized today, began to take shape in Scotland during the Middle Ages. The first written record of golf in Scotland dates back to the 15th century. The word "golf" itself is thought to have originated from the Dutch word "kolf," which means "club."

The earliest golf courses were often located on natural terrain, such as coastal sand dunes. Players would aim for specific targets, like natural holes or landmarks, rather than holes with defined numbers.

As golf grew in popularity, it became necessary to establish standardized rules. The first known written rules of golf were drafted by the Gentlemen Golfers of Edinburgh (later known as the Honourable Company of Edinburgh Golfers) in 1744. These rules laid the foundation for the modern game.

Rules of Golf

Objective: The objective of golf is to complete a course with as few strokes as possible, getting the ball from the tee (the starting point) into the hole in the fewest number of shots.

Starting Play: Golfers begin at the tee box, where they tee up their ball. The order of play is determined by the lowest score on the previous hole, with the player with the lowest score teeing off first.

Strokes: Each shot taken to advance the ball is called a "stroke." Penalty strokes are incurred for rule violations or lost balls.

Holes: Golf courses consist of 18 holes, and each hole has a designated par score, which represents the number of strokes an expert golfer should take to complete the hole.

Out of Bounds: Areas beyond the course boundaries are considered "out of bounds." Hitting the ball out of bounds results in a penalty, and the player must replay the shot.

Hazards: Hazards include bunkers (sand traps) and water hazards (lakes, ponds, streams). Players must navigate these obstacles, with specific rules for each.

Putting: On the putting green (the area surrounding the hole), players use a putter to roll the ball into the hole. The goal is to complete each hole with the fewest putts.

Etiquette: Golf has a strong emphasis on sportsmanship and etiquette, including maintaining pace of play, repairing divots and ball marks, and being considerate of other players.

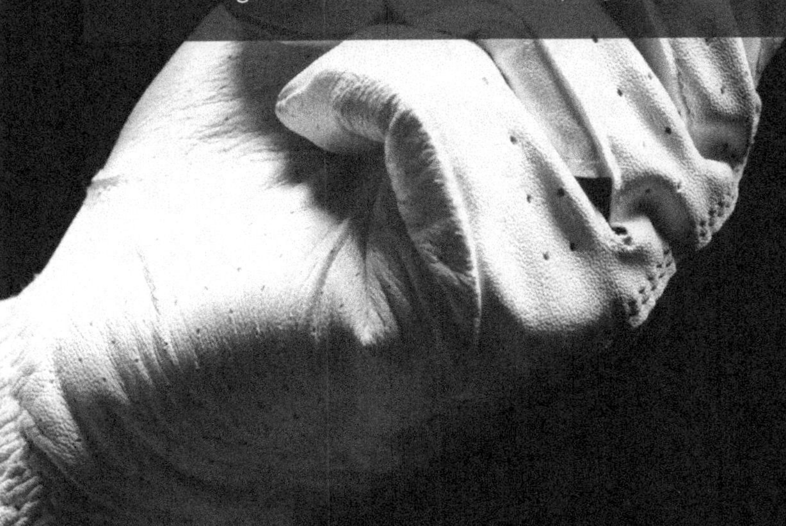

Common Golf Terms

Par: The number of strokes an expert golfer is expected to take to complete a hole.

Birdie: Completing a hole in one stroke under par.

Eagle: Completing a hole in two strokes under par.

Bogey: Completing a hole in one stroke over par.

Double Bogey: Completing a hole in two strokes over par.

Tee Box: The starting point for each hole, marked with markers for different skill levels.

Fairway: The mowed area between the tee and the green where golfers aim to hit their tee shots.

Rough: The longer grass surrounding the fairway, making it more challenging to hit accurate shots.

Green: The finely maintained area surrounding the hole where putting takes place.

Bunker: A sand trap that golfers try to avoid or escape when their ball lands in it.

Types of Golf Clubs

Driver: The longest club, used off the tee for maximum distance.
Fairway Woods: Used for long shots from the fairway or tee when the ball is sitting on the ground.

Irons: Numbered from 1 to 9, irons are used for a variety of shots, with lower-numbered irons providing more distance and higher-numbered irons offering more loft.

Wedges: Specialized irons with high lofts, used for short approach shots and getting out of bunkers.

Putter: Used on the green for putting strokes.

CRASH COURSE ON BASKETBALL

A Very Brief History Lesson

The first game was played with a soccer ball and two peach baskets as goals. The objective was to throw a soccer ball into the opposing team's basket to score points.

Basic Rules of Basketball

Team Composition: A standard basketball team consists of five players on the court at any given time. Teams can have more players on their roster, but only five can play simultaneously.

Game Duration: A regulation basketball game is typically divided into four quarters, each lasting 12 minutes (NBA) or 10 minutes (college basketball). Overtime periods may be played if the game is tied at the end of regulation.

Scoring: Points are awarded for making field goals (baskets) and free throws. A field goal made from beyond the three-point line is worth three points, while shots from inside the three-point line are worth two points. Free throws are worth one point each.

Dribbling: Players must dribble the ball (bounce it while moving) to advance it up the court. Once a player stops dribbling, they cannot resume until another player has touched the ball.

Traveling: Traveling occurs when a player takes too many steps without dribbling. It results in a turnover, with the opposing team gaining possession of the ball.

Double Dribble: A double dribble is called when a player dribbles with both hands simultaneously or starts a new dribble after stopping. It's also a turnover.

Shot Clock: In most organized basketball games, there is a shot clock, typically set to 24 seconds (NBA) or 30 seconds (college), which requires a team to attempt a shot within that time. Failing to do so results in a turnover.

Fouls: Fouls are called for various violations, such as illegal physical contact with an opponent (personal foul) or violating certain rules (e.g., goaltending). When a team accumulates a certain number of team fouls in a quarter or half, the opposing team may be awarded free throws.

Jump Ball: The game begins with a jump ball, where the referee tosses the ball into the air, and one player from each team jumps to try to catch it. The team that wins the jump ball gains the initial possession.

Common Basketball Terms:

Fast Break: An offensive play in which a team quickly moves the ball up the court to create a scoring opportunity before the opposing defense can set up.

Pick and Roll: An offensive tactic in which one player sets a screen (pick) for a ball-handler and then rolls to the basket, creating scoring opportunities.

Crossover Dribble: A dribbling move in which a player quickly changes the ball from one hand to the other to evade a defender.

Alley-Oop: A play where a player throws the ball near the basket, and a teammate jumps to catch it mid-air and score in one motion.

Rebound: When a player retrieves the ball after a missed shot.

Assist: When a player passes the ball to a teammate, leading to a made basket.

Block: When a player jumps to deflect or block an opponent's shot attempt.

Steal: When a defensive player legally takes the ball away from an offensive player, resulting in a change of possession.

Double Team: When two defensive players simultaneously guard the same offensive player to prevent them from scoring.

Triple-Double: When a player records double-digit figures (at least 10) in three statistical categories (usually points, rebounds, and assists) in a single game.

CRASH COURSE ON VOLLEYBALL

VOLLEYBALL IS 10% LUCK AND 90% BEING IN THE RIGHT PLACE AT THE RIGHT TIME.

A Very Brief History Lesson

Originally called "Mintonette," the game was designed as a recreational activity for businessmen, focusing on teamwork, cooperation, and friendly competition.

It was created as an indoor activity that combined elements of basketball, baseball, tennis, and handball to provide a less physically demanding alternative.

Basic Rules of Volleyball

Teams: Volleyball is typically played with two teams, each consisting of six players on the court at a time. However, variations with fewer players are also common.

Scoring: Volleyball is played in sets, and the team that scores 25 points first wins a set. A team must win by a margin of at least two points. If the match reaches a fifth set (in some formats), it is played to 15 points.

Rotation: Players must rotate positions clockwise each time their team wins the serve from the opposing team. This ensures that all players have an opportunity to serve and play in different positions on the court.

Serving: A point begins with a serve from behind the back boundary line (the end line). The server must strike the ball over the net into the opponent's court. The serve must clear the net and land in the opponent's court to be considered legal.

Rally Scoring: In most modern formats of volleyball, every rally (each play) results in a point, regardless of which team served. This means that a point can be won by either the serving or receiving team.

Blocking: Players can jump at the net to block an opponent's attack, but they must not interfere with the ball before or during the attacker's hit.

Three Hits: A team is allowed a maximum of three hits (contacts) to return the ball over the net: a bump (forearm pass), a set (overhead pass), and a spike (attack). Consecutive hits by the same player are not allowed.

Out-of-Bounds: The ball is considered out if it lands outside the court boundary lines or touches any object outside the court, such as the ceiling or walls.

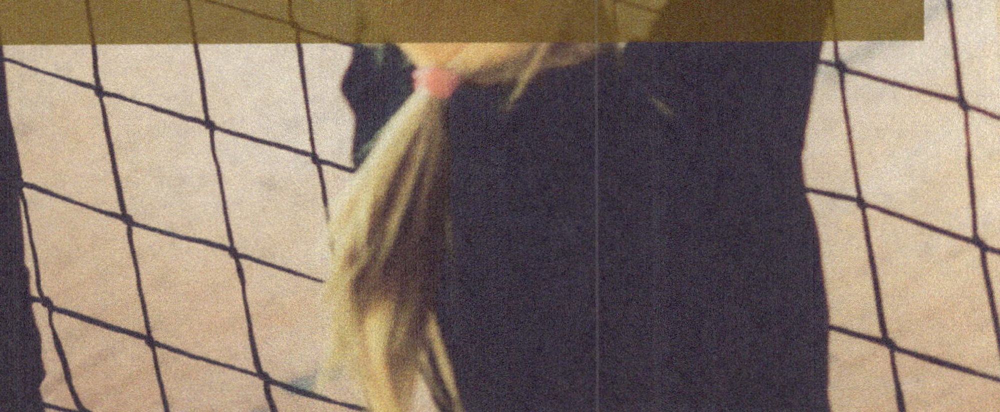

Common Volleyball Terms

Serve: The act of starting a point by hitting the ball over the net from behind the end line.

Attack: An offensive play where a player attempts to score a point by spiking or hitting the ball into the opponent's court.

Dig: A defensive play where a player dives or uses their arms to pass the ball after an opponent's attack.

Block: The act of jumping near the net to intercept an opponent's attack and prevent it from crossing the net.

Set: A high, precise pass used to set up an attacker for a spike.
Spike: A powerful downward hit used to attack and score points.

Libero: A specialized defensive player who wears a different jersey and has specific rules, such as not being allowed to serve, attack the ball above net height, or block.

Side Out: When the receiving team wins the point and earns the right to serve.

Rotation Error: A mistake that occurs when players are not in the correct rotational order, resulting in a point awarded to the opposing team.
Net Violation: A fault that occurs when a player touches the net during play.

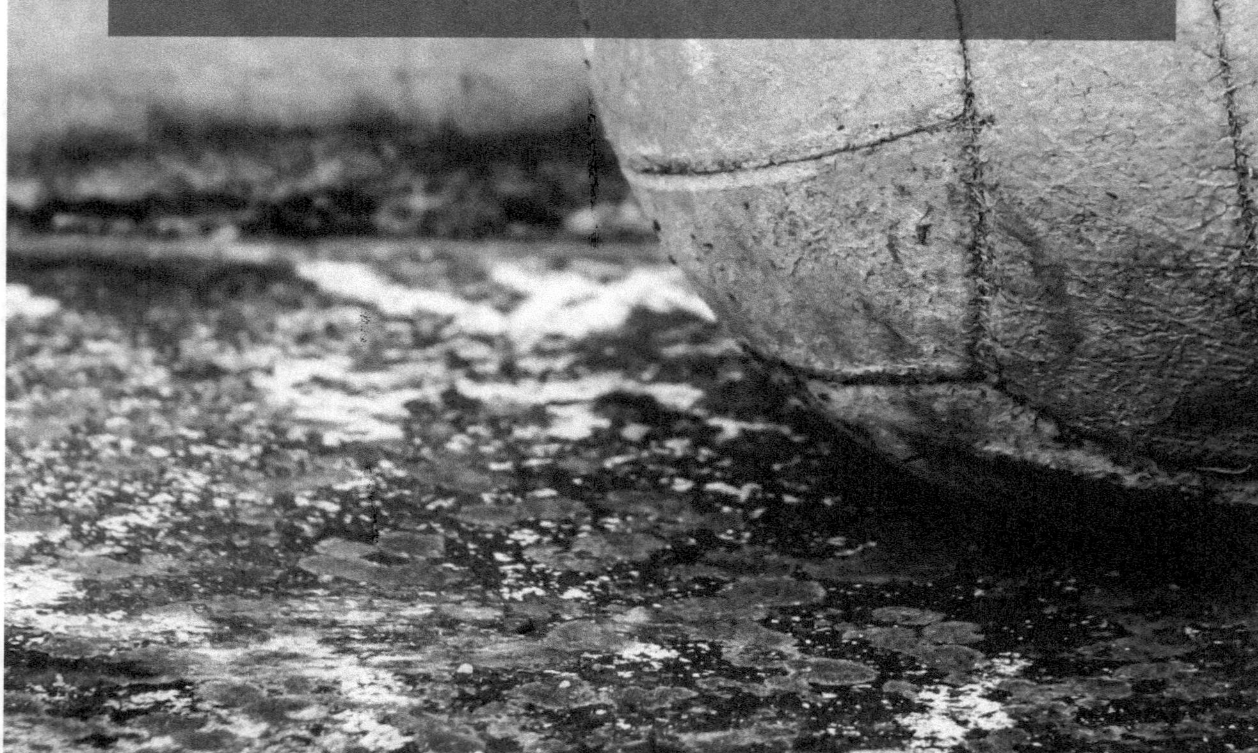

CRASH COURSE ON HOCKEY

HOCKEY IS A UNIQUE SPORT IN THE SENSE THAT YOU NEED EACH AND EVERY GUY HELPING EACH OTHER AND PULLING IN THE SAME DIRECTION TO BE SUCCESSFUL.

-Wayne Gretzky

A Brief History Lesson

The origins of hockey can be traced back to ancient civilizations, where games involving a ball and stick were played on ice or grass.

In the 19th century, field hockey gained popularity in Europe, particularly in England, where the modern rules of the game were codified.

The development of ice hockey is often credited to Canada in the 19th century. It evolved from various stick-and-ball games played on frozen ponds and rivers.

Ice Hockey Rules

Teams: Each team consists of six players on the ice at a time: three forwards, two defensemen, and a goaltender.

Scoring: Goals are scored by shooting the puck into the opponent's net. The team with the most goals at the end of the game wins.

Offsides: Players cannot enter the offensive zone (the opponent's half of the rink) ahead of the puck. If they do, it results in an offsides violation, and play is stopped.

Icing: Icing occurs when a player shoots the puck from behind the center red line across the opponent's goal line. If an opponent touches the puck first, icing is called, and play is brought back to the defensive zone of the offending team.

Penalties: Various infractions can lead to penalties, such as tripping, slashing, or high-sticking. The penalized player serves time in the penalty box, and their team plays shorthanded until the penalty time expires.

Power Play: When a team has more players on the ice due to an opponent's penalty, they are on a power play and have an advantage in trying to score.

Face-off: Play is often restarted with a face-off, where the puck is dropped between two opposing players who try to gain possession.

Blue Lines: Blue lines divide the rink into zones. Players must exit the offensive zone entirely before re-entering to avoid being offsides.

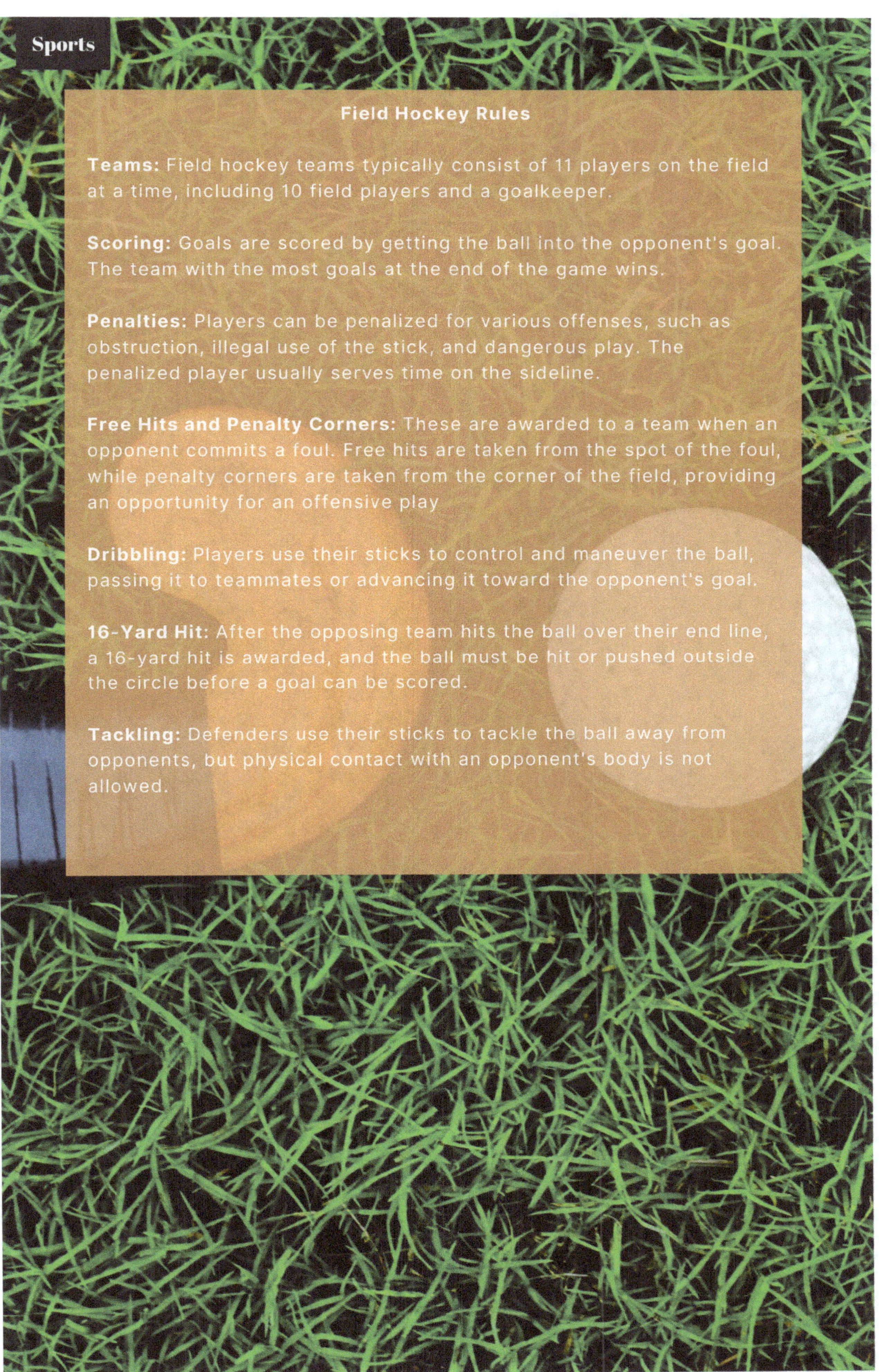

Field Hockey Rules

Teams: Field hockey teams typically consist of 11 players on the field at a time, including 10 field players and a goalkeeper.

Scoring: Goals are scored by getting the ball into the opponent's goal. The team with the most goals at the end of the game wins.

Penalties: Players can be penalized for various offenses, such as obstruction, illegal use of the stick, and dangerous play. The penalized player usually serves time on the sideline.

Free Hits and Penalty Corners: These are awarded to a team when an opponent commits a foul. Free hits are taken from the spot of the foul, while penalty corners are taken from the corner of the field, providing an opportunity for an offensive play

Dribbling: Players use their sticks to control and maneuver the ball, passing it to teammates or advancing it toward the opponent's goal.

16-Yard Hit: After the opposing team hits the ball over their end line, a 16-yard hit is awarded, and the ball must be hit or pushed outside the circle before a goal can be scored.

Tackling: Defenders use their sticks to tackle the ball away from opponents, but physical contact with an opponent's body is not allowed.

Common Hockey Terms (Both Ice and Field)

Stickhandling: Skillful use of the stick to control and maneuver the puck or ball.

Forecheck: Defensive players pressure the opposing team in their offensive zone to disrupt their play.

Backcheck: Players hustle back to their own defensive zone to prevent the opponent from scoring on a counterattack.

Breakaway: A situation where an offensive player has a clear path to the opponent's goal with no defenders between them and the goaltender.

Crease: The marked area in front of the goal where the goaltender is stationed; offensive players are not allowed to enter this area.

Power Forward: A player known for their physicality and scoring ability.

Hat Trick: Scoring three goals in a single game.

Top Shelf: Refers to scoring a goal by shooting the puck or ball into the top part of the net.

CRASH COURSE ON BASEBALL

BASEBALL IS NINETY PERCENT MENTAL AND THE OTHER HALF IS PHYSICAL.

- Yogi Berra

A Brief History Lesson

Baseball's origins are somewhat debated, but it is believed to have evolved from older bat-and-ball games played in England (Cricket).

The story of Abner Doubleday inventing baseball in Cooperstown, New York, in 1839 is a popular myth but not historically accurate. Baseball's development was a gradual process, and no single individual can be credited with inventing the game.

Basic Rules of Baseball

Teams: Baseball is played between two teams, each consisting of nine players. One team bats while the other team fields. The roles switch after each half-inning.

Innings: A standard baseball game is divided into nine innings, with each team taking turns batting and fielding. If the game is tied after nine innings, extra innings are played until a winner is determined.

Scoring: The objective for the batting team is to score runs by having their players cross home plate. Runs are scored when a batter hits the ball and reaches base safely while other runners advance around the bases and cross home plate.

Pitching: The pitcher is the player who throws the ball to the batter from the pitcher's mound. The pitcher tries to strike out the batter (get three strikes) or induce them to hit the ball to the fielders.

Bases: There are four bases in baseball: first, second, third, and home plate. Runners advance from base to base in a counter-clockwise direction.

Outs: Each team gets three outs per inning while batting. An out can occur in various ways, such as a strikeout, a caught fly ball, a force play, or a tag out.

Baserunning: Runners must stay in contact with the base until the pitcher delivers the ball. They can advance when the pitcher pitches the ball and when a batter hits the ball safely into play.

Foul Balls: A batted ball that lands outside the foul lines is called a foul ball. Foul balls count as strikes unless a batter already has two strikes.

Home Run: When a batter hits the ball out of the playing field, it's called a home run, and the batter and any other runners on base score automatically.

Extra Bases: Batters can advance more than one base on a single hit, such as a double (advancing to second base), a triple (to third base), or an inside-the-park home run.

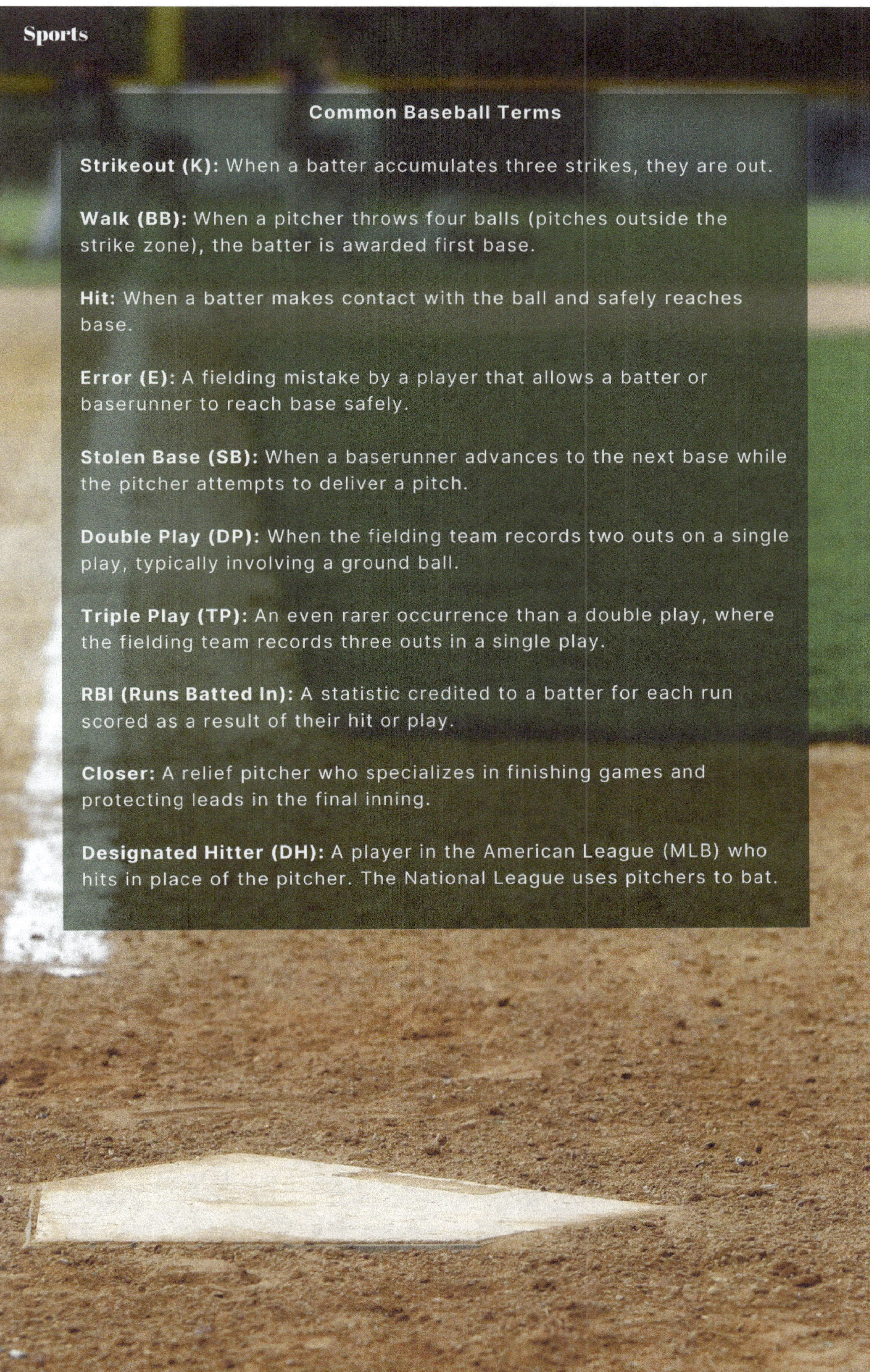

Common Baseball Terms

Strikeout (K): When a batter accumulates three strikes, they are out.

Walk (BB): When a pitcher throws four balls (pitches outside the strike zone), the batter is awarded first base.

Hit: When a batter makes contact with the ball and safely reaches base.

Error (E): A fielding mistake by a player that allows a batter or baserunner to reach base safely.

Stolen Base (SB): When a baserunner advances to the next base while the pitcher attempts to deliver a pitch.

Double Play (DP): When the fielding team records two outs on a single play, typically involving a ground ball.

Triple Play (TP): An even rarer occurrence than a double play, where the fielding team records three outs in a single play.

RBI (Runs Batted In): A statistic credited to a batter for each run scored as a result of their hit or play.

Closer: A relief pitcher who specializes in finishing games and protecting leads in the final inning.

Designated Hitter (DH): A player in the American League (MLB) who hits in place of the pitcher. The National League uses pitchers to bat.

CRASH COURSE ON RUGBY

SOCCER IS A GENTLEMAN'S GAME PLAYED BY HOOLIGANS, AND RUGBY IS A HOOLIGAN'S GAME PLAYED BY GENTLEMEN.

A Brief History Lesson

Rugby's origins can be traced back to England in the early 19th century. The precise origins are somewhat debated, but it is generally believed to have evolved from various forms of football (soccer) that were played in schools and communities.

In 1823, a defining moment in rugby history occurred when a young man named William Webb Ellis is said to have picked up the ball during a game of soccer at Rugby School and ran with it, essentially creating a new style of play. This act is often credited with giving rise to rugby football.

Basic Rules of Rugby

Objective: The primary goal in rugby is to carry, pass, or kick the ball across the opponent's goal line and touch it down to score points.

Teams: Rugby is played with two teams, each consisting of 15 players (in rugby union) or 13 players (in rugby league) on the field at a time.

Scoring: Points can be scored in several ways:
- A "try" is worth 5 points and is scored by touching the ball down in the opponent's in-goal area.
- A "conversion" is worth 2 points and is attempted by kicking the ball through the goalposts after a try.
- A "penalty goal" is worth 3 points and is awarded for certain rule violations.
- A "drop goal" is worth 3 points and is scored by kicking the ball through the goalposts during open play.

Ball Handling: Players can pass the ball laterally or backward to teammates but cannot pass it forward. The ball can be kicked or carried, but players cannot use their hands or arms to pass it forward.

Tackling: Tackling is a fundamental part of rugby. Players can tackle opponents by grabbing them below the shoulders and pulling them to the ground. Dangerous tackles or high tackles are penalized.

Rucks and Mauls: When a player is tackled and brought to the ground, a ruck or maul may form. In a ruck, players from both teams compete for the ball on the ground. In a maul, players bind together while on their feet, with the ball at the center.

Lineouts and Scrums: Lineouts occur when the ball goes out of bounds, and teams compete to catch a throw-in from the touchline. Scrums are contested formations that restart play after certain infringements, with players from both teams engaging in a pushing contest to win the ball.

Offside Rule: Players must stay behind the ball when it is kicked, passed, or carried by their teammates. Being in an offside position can result in a penalty.

Common Rugby Terms

Forward: Players in the forward positions are typically involved in the physical aspects of the game, such as scrums, rucks, and mauls.

Back: Players in the back positions are usually faster and more skilled at handling the ball, often involved in running, passing, and kicking.

Try: Scoring a try is the primary way to earn points in rugby. It involves touching the ball down in the opponent's in-goal area.

Conversion: After a try is scored, a conversion attempt is taken by kicking the ball through the goalposts. Successful conversions add two points to the team's score.

Penalty: When a rule is violated, the opposing team may be awarded a penalty. They can choose to kick the ball for a penalty goal attempt or use it to restart play.

Scrum: A method of restarting play after certain stoppages, involving a contested formation of players from both teams binding together and trying to win the ball.

Ruck: A contest for possession that occurs on the ground after a tackle, with players from both teams attempting to secure the ball.

Maul: Similar to a ruck, but players remain on their feet and bind together while trying to move forward with the ball.

Lineout: A method of restarting play after the ball goes out of bounds, with players competing to catch a throw-in from the touchline.

Drop Goal: A field goal attempt taken during open play by kicking the ball through the goalposts.

CRASH COURSE ON CRICKET

IT'S NOT WHETHER YOU GET KNOCKED DOWN, IT'S WHETHER YOU GET UP.

-Sir Vivian Richards

A Brief History Lesson

The exact origins of cricket are not entirely clear, but it is believed to have evolved in England during the late 16th century.

The Ashes series, one of cricket's most iconic rivalries, began in 1882 when Australia defeated England at The Oval in London. A mock obituary in The Sporting Times stated that English cricket had died, and "the body will be cremated and the ashes taken to Australia."

Basic Rules of Cricket

Teams: Cricket is typically played between two teams, with each team consisting of 11 players.

Overs: The game is divided into "overs," each consisting of six deliveries (bowled by the same bowler). The number of overs in a match can vary, with common formats being T20 (20 overs per side), One Day International (ODI, 50 overs per side), and Test cricket (unlimited overs over five days).

Pitch: Cricket is played on a rectangular field with a strip of closely trimmed grass called the "pitch" at the center. There are two sets of stumps (three wooden sticks) at each end of the pitch, with bails placed on top of the stumps.

Batting: One team bats while the other team bowls and fields. The batting team aims to score runs by hitting the ball and running between the wickets or hitting boundaries (four runs for the ball reaching the boundary, and six runs for hitting it over the boundary).

Bowling: The bowling team tries to dismiss the batsmen by getting them out through various means, such as getting them bowled (hitting the stumps with the ball), caught (fielder catches the ball), LBW (leg before wicket, when the ball would have hit the stumps but for the player's leg obstructing it), and more.

Fielding: The fielding team aims to prevent the batting team from scoring runs and taking wickets by fielding the ball and trying to dismiss batsmen.

Scoring: Runs are scored by running between the wickets or hitting boundaries. A single run is scored when the batsmen run from one end to the other. Batsmen can also score "extras" through no-balls (an illegal delivery), wides (balls bowled too wide of the stumps), and byes (runs scored when the ball passes the batsman without contact).

Wickets: The set of stumps at each end is referred to as a "wicket." Dismissing a batsman by hitting the stumps or through other means is known as taking a "wicket."

Common Cricket Terms

Innings: A team's turn to bat and field. In limited-overs cricket (T20, ODI), each team gets one innings, while in Test cricket, teams have two innings each.

Bowler: A player who delivers the ball to the batsman.

Batsman: A player from the batting team who faces the bowler's deliveries.

Captain: The leader of each cricket team who makes strategic decisions on the field.

Umpire: The officials responsible for enforcing the rules and making decisions on the field.

Run Rate: The average number of runs scored per over.

Duck: When a batsman is dismissed without scoring any runs in an innings, it is referred to as getting a "duck."

Boundary: The outer edge of the cricket field where a four (ball reaching the boundary) or six (ball going over the boundary) is scored.

Spinner: A type of bowler who specializes in spinning the ball to deceive the batsman. Common spin deliveries include the off-spin and leg-spin.

Fast Bowler: A bowler who delivers the ball at high speeds, often generating bounce and swing.

CRASH COURSE ON AMERICAN FOOTBALL

FOOTBALL IS NOT A CONTACT SPORT; IT'S A COLLISION SPORT. DANCING IS A CONTACT SPORT.

-Vince Lombardi

A Brief History Lesson

American football evolved from a combination of rugby and soccer, both of which were popular in the United States in the mid-19th century.

The game started to take shape in the 1860s and 1870s, with colleges and universities developing their own variations of football with different rules.

The introduction of the forward pass in the early 20th century by quarterback John Wesley "Pop" Warner and others revolutionized the game. Previously, only lateral or backward passes were allowed.

This change made the game more open and dynamic, leading to the development of the passing game.

Basic Rules of American Football

Team Composition: Each team consists of 11 players on the field at a time, divided into offense and defense. Teams can have a larger roster, but only 11 players are allowed on the field simultaneously.

Scoring: Teams score points by advancing the ball into the opposing team's end zone or by kicking the ball through the opponent's goalposts.

The Field: The football field is 100 yards long and 53.3 yards wide. It is marked with yard lines, hash marks, and end zones.

Play Duration: A standard American football game is divided into four quarters, each lasting 15 minutes. Overtime periods may be played if the game is tied at the end of regulation.

Offense: The offensive team tries to advance the ball down the field to score. They have four downs (attempts) to advance at least 10 yards. If they succeed, they get another set of four downs.

Defense: The defensive team tries to prevent the offense from advancing the ball and scoring. They aim to tackle the ball carrier, intercept passes, or force fumbles.

Scrimmage: Each play begins with a snap from the center to the quarterback. The line of scrimmage is the imaginary line where the ball is placed before the snap.

Touchdown: The primary way to score in football is by carrying the ball across the opponent's goal line or catching a pass in the end zone, resulting in a touchdown worth six points.

Field Goal: A field goal is worth three points and is scored by successfully kicking the ball through the opponent's goalposts.

Extra Point: After a touchdown, the scoring team has the option to kick an extra point (worth one point) or attempt a two-point conversion (worth two points) from a closer distance.

Common American Football Terms

Quarterback (QB): The leader of the offense, responsible for passing the ball and making decisions during plays.

Running Back (RB): A player who carries the ball and runs with it.

Wide Receiver (WR): A player who catches passes from the quarterback.

Tight End (TE): A player who serves as both a blocker and a receiver.

Offensive Line (OL): The group of players responsible for protecting the quarterback and creating running lanes.

Line of Scrimmage: The imaginary line where the ball is placed before each play.

Interception: When a defensive player catches a pass intended for an offensive player.

Sack: When the quarterback is tackled behind the line of scrimmage before he can throw the ball.

Fumble: When a player drops the ball while running or being tackled, resulting in a live ball that can be recovered by either team.

Blitz: A defensive strategy where additional players rush the quarterback in an attempt to disrupt the play.

Punt: A kick used to give possession to the opposing team while maximizing the field position.

CRASH COURSE ON FOOTBALL / SOCCER

THE BEAUTIFUL GAME

A Brief History Lesson

The roots of soccer can be traced back to ancient civilizations. Various cultures, including the Greeks, Romans, Chinese, and Indigenous peoples of Mesoamerica, played games involving a ball and feet.

Mob football, for example, was a rough and chaotic form of football played in medieval England, where entire villages would compete against each other in a frenzied manner.

The sport's simplicity and low equipment requirements made it accessible and attractive to people of all ages and backgrounds.

Basic Rules of Soccer

Teams: Each team consists of 11 players, including a goalkeeper and outfield players. Teams may have substitutes who can replace players during the match.

Field of Play: Soccer is played on a rectangular field with specific dimensions. The field is marked with lines, including the touchlines (sidelines) and goal lines.

Duration: A standard soccer match consists of two halves, each lasting 45 minutes. There is a 15-minute halftime break between the halves. In some competitions, extra time and penalty shootouts may be used to determine a winner if the match ends in a tie.

Scoring: The objective is to score goals by getting the ball into the opponent's goal. Each goal is worth one point.

Offside: The offside rule prevents players from positioning themselves behind the last defender (excluding the goalkeeper) at the moment the ball is played to them. Being offside results in a free-kick for the opposing team.

Fouls and Free Kicks: Fouls are committed when a player engages in prohibited actions, such as tripping, pushing, or handling the ball with their hands (except for the goalkeeper within the penalty area). Fouls result in free kicks for the opposing team.

Penalty Kick: A penalty kick is awarded when a foul occurs inside the penalty area. It involves a one-on-one situation between the attacking player and the goalkeeper from the penalty spot.

Throw-in: When the ball goes out of bounds over the touchline, the opposing team is awarded a throw-in. The player taking the throw-in must have both feet on the ground and use a two-handed throw.

Goal Kick: When the attacking team kicks the ball out of bounds over the goal line, the defending team is awarded a goal kick. The ball is placed in the six-yard box and kicked back into play.

Corner Kick: If the defending team kicks the ball out of bounds over the goal line, the attacking team is awarded a corner kick. The ball is placed in the corner arc and then played into the penalty area.

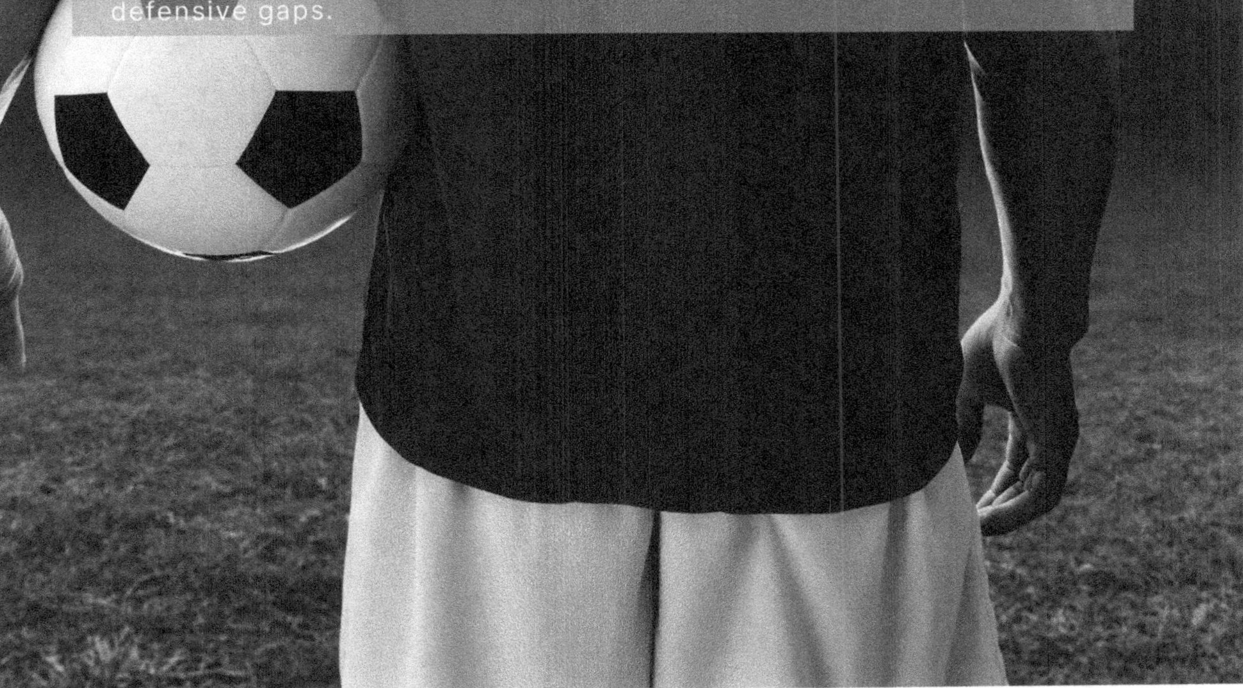

Common Soccer Terms

Dribbling: The act of controlling the ball while running or walking to move it past opponents.

Pass: A deliberate kick or header to transfer the ball to a teammate.

Tackle: An attempt to take the ball away from an opponent's possession, often involving sliding or using the feet to dispossess the opponent.

Header: Using the head to direct or pass the ball.

Nutmeg: A move where a player passes the ball through an opponent's legs and regains possession.

Booking: When a player receives a yellow card (caution) or a red card (expulsion) for committing fouls or unsportsmanlike behavior.

Hat-Trick: When a player scores three goals in a single game.

Injury Time (Added Time): Additional time added to each half to compensate for stoppages and delays during the match.

Counterattack: A fast-paced offensive play where a team quickly transitions from defense to attack to catch the opposing team off guard.

Sweeper: A defensive player who plays behind the main line of defenders and is responsible for clearing the ball and covering defensive gaps.

CRASH COURSE ON BADMINTON

BADMINTON IS LIKE BALLET DANCING. IT REQUIRES A LOT OF CONTROL, STRENGTH, MIND PLAY, AND MEASURED MOVEMENT.

A Brief History Lesson

Badminton has its roots in ancient civilizations, with games that involved hitting a shuttlecock or birdie (a projectile with feathers) back and forth with various objects.

The earliest known version of the game was called "Poona" or "Poonah," named after a British garrison town in India where British Army officers stationed there in the mid-19th century adapted and popularized the game.

Basic Rules of Badminton

Scoring: Badminton is played in sets, and a match is typically the best of three sets. Each set is played to 21 points, with a margin of two points required to win. If the score reaches 20-20, the set continues until one player/team has a two-point lead.

Serving: The server must stand within their service court (a diagonal box marked on the court) and hit the shuttlecock diagonally over the net into the opponent's service court. The serve must be underhand and below the waist.

Scoring System: Only the serving side can score points. If the serving side wins a rally, they score a point and continue to serve. If the receiving side wins a rally, they gain the serve but do not score a point.

Doubles Rules: In doubles, each team has two players. The server must serve diagonally to the opposing team's service court, and the receiving team must decide which player will receive the serve.

Faults: Common faults include serving or hitting the shuttlecock outside the boundaries, letting the shuttlecock hit the ground, obstructing the opponent's view, and making illegal contact with the net or the shuttlecock.

Common Badminton Terms

Shuttlecock: The feathered or synthetic projectile that is hit back and forth over the net.

Rally: A sequence of shots or exchanges between players until the point is won or lost.

Service Court: The designated area where a player must stand to serve the shuttlecock.

Fault: An infringement of the rules, which results in the loss of a point or the serve.

Smash: A powerful overhead shot where the player hits the shuttlecock steeply downward into the opponent's court.

Drop Shot: A softly hit shot that barely clears the net and lands close to the net on the opponent's side.

Clear: A high, deep shot that sends the shuttlecock to the back of the opponent's court, used to create space or gain time.

Drive: A fast, flat shot that travels horizontally over the net, used for aggressive play.

Net Shot: A shot that is played softly and close to the net, often used to deceive the opponent.

Deuce: A term used when the score is tied at 20-20, requiring one side to win by a margin of two points to claim the set.

Match Point: The point that could potentially win the match if the player/team wins it.

Game Point: The point that could potentially win the game or set if the player/team wins it.

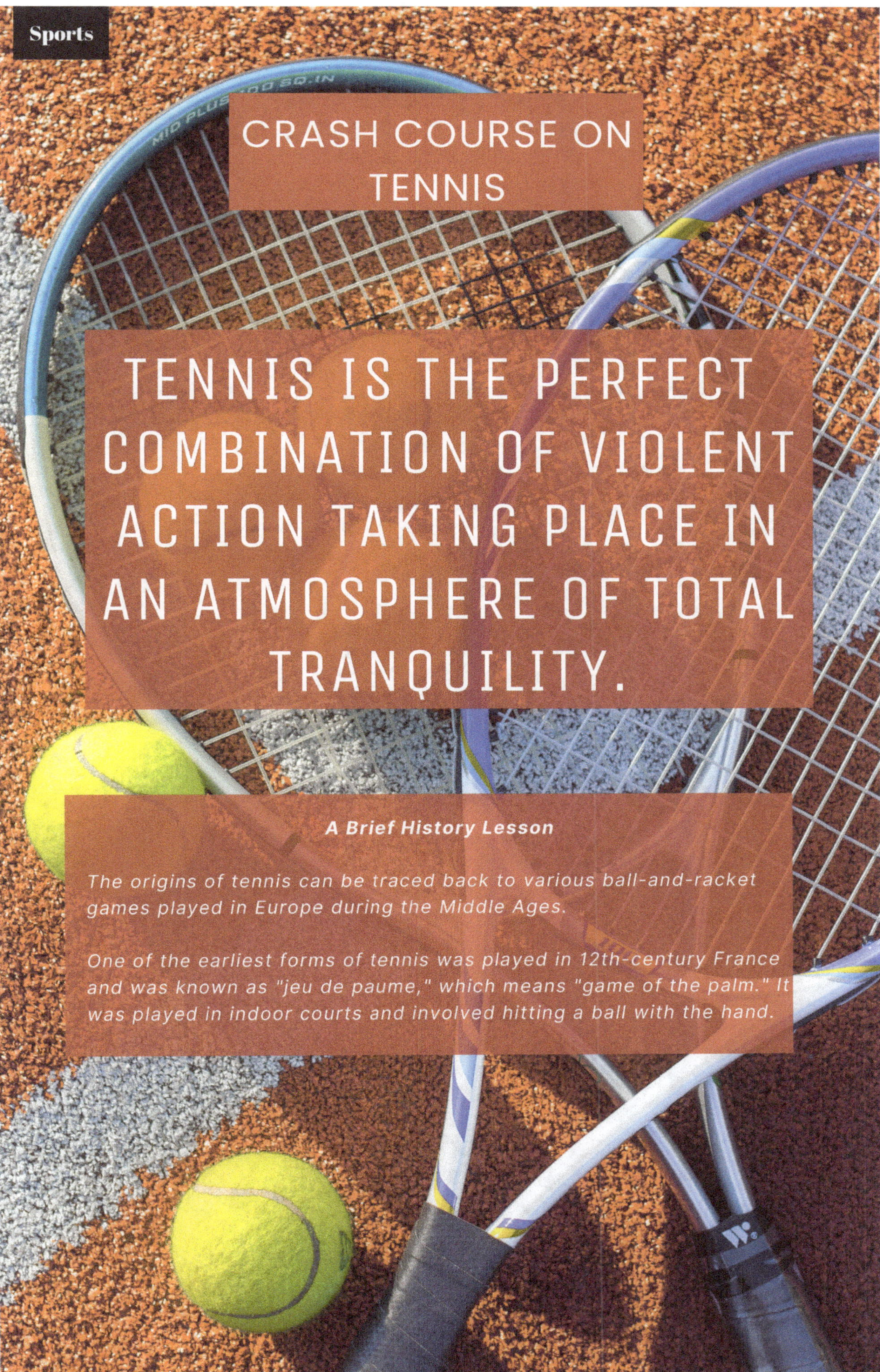

CRASH COURSE ON TENNIS

TENNIS IS THE PERFECT COMBINATION OF VIOLENT ACTION TAKING PLACE IN AN ATMOSPHERE OF TOTAL TRANQUILITY.

A Brief History Lesson

The origins of tennis can be traced back to various ball-and-racket games played in Europe during the Middle Ages.

One of the earliest forms of tennis was played in 12th-century France and was known as "jeu de paume," which means "game of the palm." It was played in indoor courts and involved hitting a ball with the hand.

Basic Rules of Tennis

Scoring System: Tennis uses a scoring system based on points, games, and sets.

- Points: The first point is called "15," the second point is "30," and the third point is "40." If both players or teams have 40 points, it's referred to as "deuce."
- Advantage: After deuce, a player must win two consecutive points to win the game.
- Games: To win a game, a player or team must win four points and have a two-point lead. The first player or team to win six games (with a two-game lead) wins the set.
- Sets: Matches are typically played as best-of-three sets or best-of-five sets (in major tournaments like Grand Slams). To win a set, a player or team must win six games with a two-game lead. If the set reaches 6-6, a tiebreaker may be played to determine the winner of the set.

Serving: Players take turns serving. The server stands behind the baseline and must serve diagonally to the opponent's service box. The server gets two attempts (first and second serve). If they fail to get the ball in play on both attempts, it's called a "double fault," and the opponent wins a point.

Scoring in a Game: The server's score is always announced first. For example, if the server wins the first point, the score is "15-0" (15 for the server, 0 for the receiver). If the receiver wins the next point, it becomes "15-15," and so on.

Court: A standard tennis court is divided into two halves by a net. The two sides are called "singles" and "doubles" courts, depending on the type of match. The lines on the court include the baseline, service line, center service line, and sidelines.

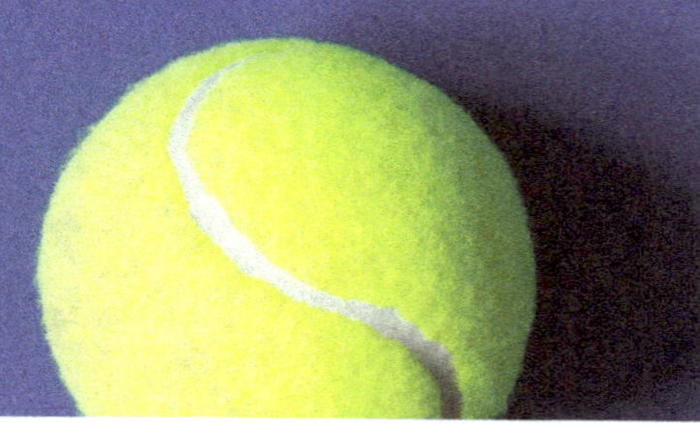

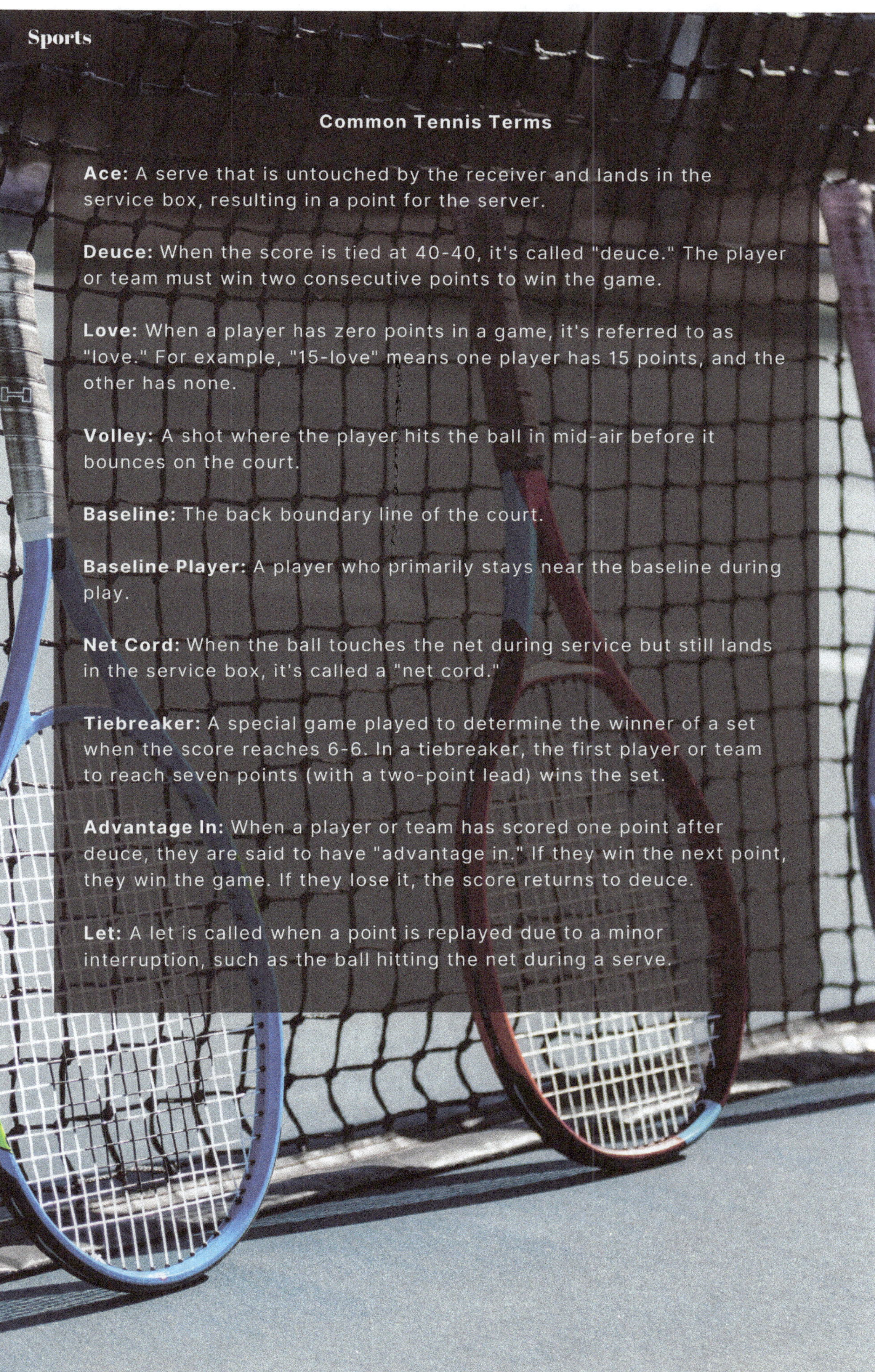

Common Tennis Terms

Ace: A serve that is untouched by the receiver and lands in the service box, resulting in a point for the server.

Deuce: When the score is tied at 40-40, it's called "deuce." The player or team must win two consecutive points to win the game.

Love: When a player has zero points in a game, it's referred to as "love." For example, "15-love" means one player has 15 points, and the other has none.

Volley: A shot where the player hits the ball in mid-air before it bounces on the court.

Baseline: The back boundary line of the court.

Baseline Player: A player who primarily stays near the baseline during play.

Net Cord: When the ball touches the net during service but still lands in the service box, it's called a "net cord."

Tiebreaker: A special game played to determine the winner of a set when the score reaches 6-6. In a tiebreaker, the first player or team to reach seven points (with a two-point lead) wins the set.

Advantage In: When a player or team has scored one point after deuce, they are said to have "advantage in." If they win the next point, they win the game. If they lose it, the score returns to deuce.

Let: A let is called when a point is replayed due to a minor interruption, such as the ball hitting the net during a serve.

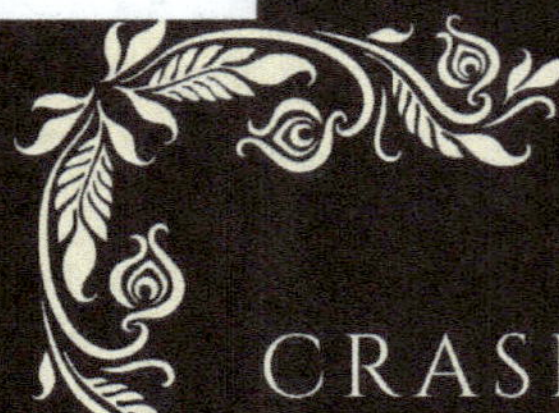

SHERLOCK

ELEMENTARY, MY DEAR WATSON

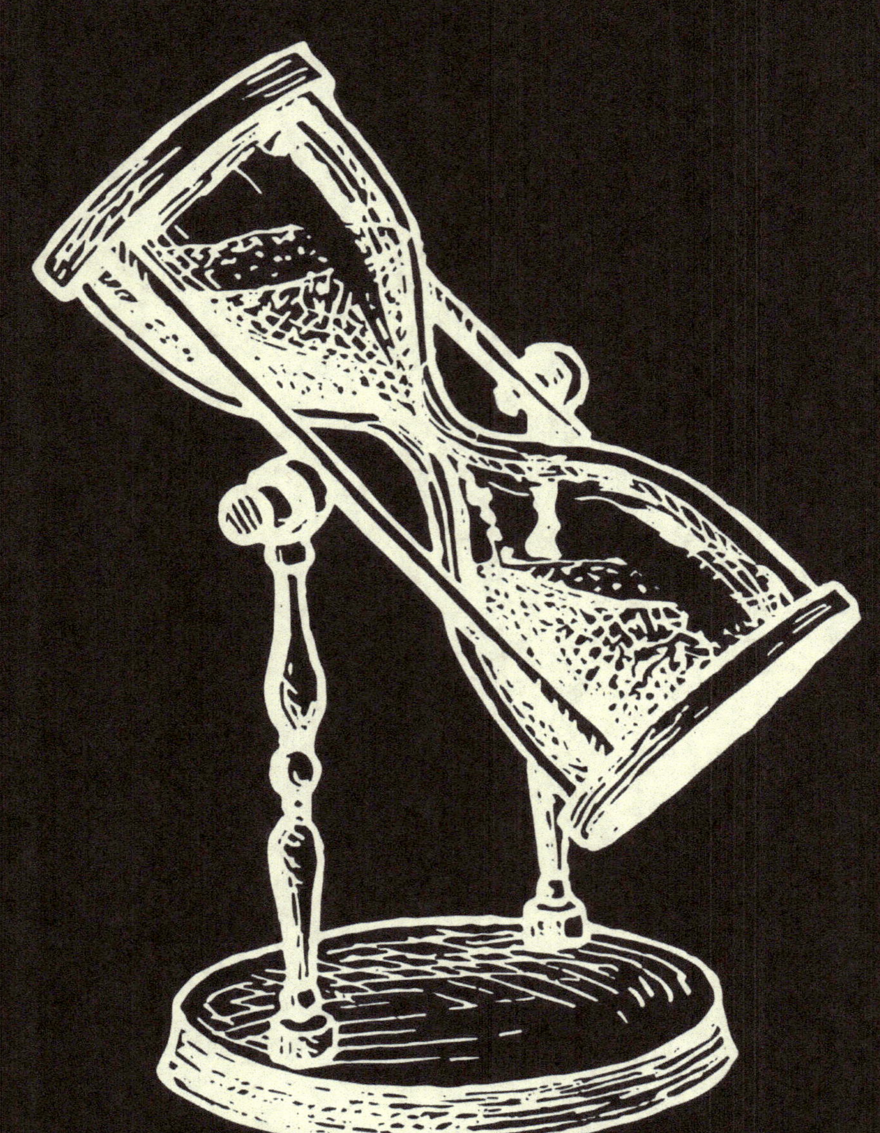

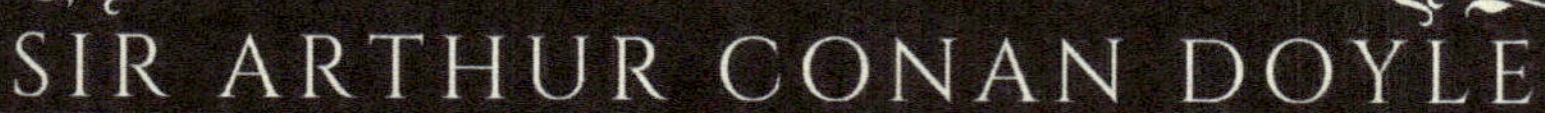

SIR ARTHUR CONAN DOYLE

Creation and Authorship:
Sherlock Holmes was created by Sir Arthur Conan Doyle, a British author and physician.
He first appeared in the novel "A Study in Scarlet," published in 1887.

Fictional Setting:
Sherlock Holmes and his loyal friend and chronicler, Dr. John H. Watson, are based in London, primarily during the late 19th and early 20th centuries, known as the Victorian and Edwardian eras.

Character Traits:
Sherlock Holmes is known for his brilliant deductive reasoning, keen observation skills, and logical thinking.
He is often described as cold, calculating, and unemotional, but also highly eccentric.
Holmes has a deep appreciation for music, plays the violin, and is skilled in chemistry and forensic science.

Residence:
Sherlock Holmes resides at 221B Baker Street in London, a fictional address that has become synonymous with his character.

Methods of Deduction:
Holmes often uses his famous catchphrase, "Elementary, my dear Watson," though this exact phrase is not found in the original stories.
His methods of deduction involve careful observation of details, logical reasoning, and an encyclopaedic knowledge of various subjects.

Nemesis:
Holmes' arch-nemesis is Professor James Moriarty, a brilliant criminal mastermind who matches Holmes' intellect.

Watson's Role:
Dr. John Watson is Holmes' loyal friend and biographer.
Watson often serves as the reader's point of view into Holmes' deductive processes and adventures.

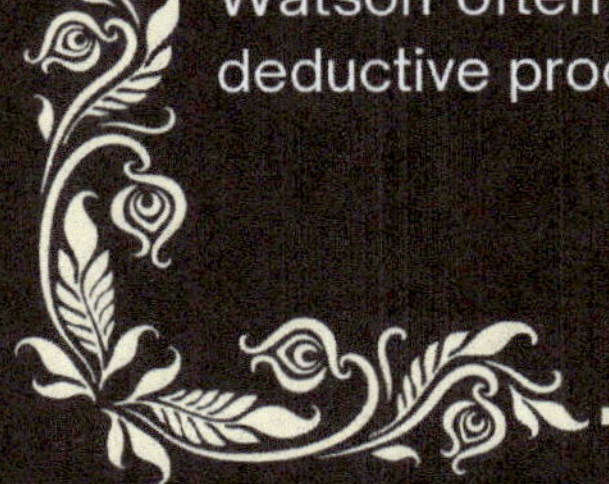

Legacy:
Sherlock Holmes has had a profound and lasting impact on popular culture and detective fiction.
Numerous adaptations, including movies, television series, and radio dramas, have been made featuring Holmes and Watson.
The character has become a symbol of deductive reasoning and the detective archetype.

Authorship Controversy:
Sir Arthur Conan Doyle initially killed off Holmes in "The Final Problem" (1893) but was compelled to resurrect him due to popular demand.
This decision led to a feud between Doyle and Holmes fans.

Holmes' Retirement:
Holmes is said to have retired to beekeeping on the Sussex Downs after faking his own death in "The Final Problem." He later returned in "The Adventure of the Empty House."

Adaptations and Pop Culture:
Sherlock Holmes has been portrayed by numerous actors, with some of the most notable being Basil Rathbone, Jeremy Brett, Robert Downey Jr., and Benedict Cumberbatch.
Modern adaptations like the BBC's "Sherlock" and the "Elementary" TV series have brought the character into contemporary settings.

Influence on Detective Fiction:
Sherlock Holmes is often considered the prototype for the modern detective in literature and has inspired countless other fictional detectives and investigators.

Famous Stories and Novels

"The Hound of the Baskervilles":

This novel is one of the most famous Sherlock Holmes stories and is set in the eerie moors of Devonshire. It revolves around the legend of a ghostly hound that haunts the Baskerville family, leading to mysterious deaths. Holmes and Watson are called to investigate the death of Sir Charles Baskerville and to protect the heir, Sir Henry Baskerville, from a similar fate. The story combines elements of the supernatural with Holmes' rational approach to uncover the truth.

"The Adventures of Sherlock Holmes" (Collection of Short Stories):

This collection contains twelve short stories, each featuring a distinct case or mystery. Some of the notable stories include:
"A Scandal in Bohemia": Holmes matches wits with Irene Adler, a talented opera singer.
"The Adventure of the Speckled Band": Holmes investigates the mysterious death of a young woman whose sister claims to have heard a strange whistling noise.
"The Red-Headed League": Holmes unravels a bizarre plot involving a secret society that targets red-headed men for a peculiar job offer.
These stories showcase Holmes' diverse range of cases and his brilliant deductive abilities.

"The Sign of Four":

In this novel, Holmes and Watson are hired to investigate a complex case involving a stolen treasure and a mysterious message involving four symbols. The story delves into the history of colonial India, treasure hunts, and a dangerous criminal seeking revenge. It also introduces Dr. John Watson to his future wife, Mary Morstan, adding a romantic subplot to the mystery.

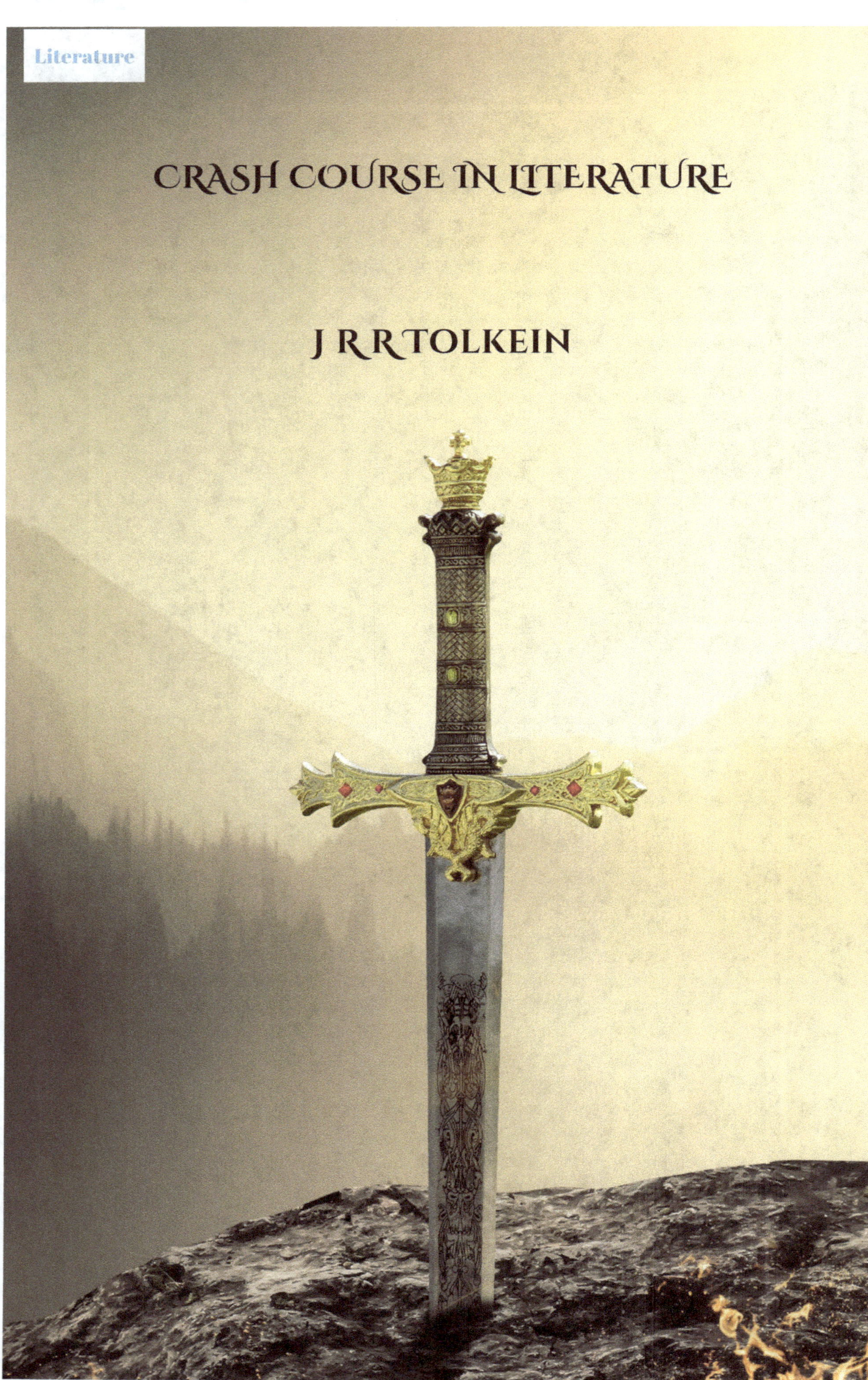
Literature
CRASH COURSE IN LITERATURE
J R R TOLKEIN

Early Life:
J.R.R. Tolkien was born on January 3, 1892, in Bloemfontein, South Africa, but he spent most of his childhood in England after his family returned there when he was three years old. His father died when he was very young, and his mother passed away when he was just twelve.

Academic Career:
Tolkien had a distinguished academic career. He studied at Exeter College, Oxford, and later became a professor of Anglo-Saxon at Pembroke College, Oxford. He also held the position of the Rawlinson and Bosworth Professor of Anglo-Saxon.

Languages:
Tolkien was a philologist with a deep interest in languages. He created several constructed languages, the most famous of which is Elvish. His passion for languages heavily influenced the creation of Middle-earth, the fictional world in which his stories are set.

The Hobbit:
Tolkien's first major work, "The Hobbit," was published in 1937. It's a fantasy novel that introduces readers to the world of Middle-earth and follows the adventures of Bilbo Baggins, a hobbit who embarks on a quest with a group of dwarves.

The Lord of the Rings: Tolkien's magnum opus, "The Lord of the Rings," is a high-fantasy epic published in three volumes between 1954 and 1955. It consists of "The Fellowship of the Ring," "The Two Towers," and "The Return of the King." The story follows the quest to destroy the One Ring and defeat the Dark Lord Sauron.

Influence:
Tolkien's works have had a profound and lasting impact on the fantasy genre. His intricate world-building, memorable characters, and epic storytelling have inspired countless authors, filmmakers, and artists.

Adaptations: "The Lord of the Rings" has been adapted into a highly successful film trilogy directed by Peter Jackson, released between 2001 and 2003. "The Hobbit" was also adapted into a film trilogy by Jackson, released between 2012 and 2014.

Quotes to Note

From "The Hobbit":

"In a hole in the ground there lived a hobbit."

"The world is indeed full of peril, and in it there are many dark places; but still there is much that is fair, and though in all lands love is now mingled with grief, it grows perhaps the greater."

From "The Lord of the Rings":

"The road goes ever on and on, down from the door where it began. Now far ahead the road has gone, and I must follow if I can."

"Even the smallest person can change the course of the future."

"I wish it need not have happened in my time," said Frodo. "So do I," said Gandalf, "and so do all who live to see such times. But that is not for them to decide. All we have to decide is what to do with the time that is given us."

"The world is indeed full of peril, and in it there are many dark places; but still there is much that is fair, and though in all lands love is now mingled with grief, it grows perhaps the greater."
"There is some good in this world, and it's worth fighting for."
"The Shadow does not hold sway yet, not over you and not over me."

KING

Stephen King is a prolific and highly influential American author known primarily for his work in the horror, supernatural fiction, and suspense genres.

Famous books with plot and dialogues to quote

"Carrie" (1974):
Plot Synopsis: "Carrie" tells the story of Carrie White, a teenage girl with telekinetic powers who is relentlessly bullied at school. When she's pushed too far, she unleashes her terrifying abilities at the prom, resulting in a bloodbath.
Movie Adaptation: The novel has been adapted into several films, with the most well-known being the 1976 version directed by Brian De Palma.

"The Shining" (1977):
Plot Synopsis: "The Shining" follows the Torrance family as they move to the isolated Overlook Hotel to serve as winter caretakers. The hotel's malevolent supernatural forces begin to affect the family, particularly Jack Torrance, who descends into madness.
Movie Adaptation: Stanley Kubrick directed a famous adaptation in 1980, and a TV miniseries adaptation was released in 1997.
Famous Dialogue: "Here's Johnny!"

"It" (1986):
Plot Synopsis: "It" is set in the fictional town of Derry, Maine, where a group of friends confront a shape-shifting entity that preys on children and often takes the form of Pennywise the Clown. They return as adults to face the evil again.
Movie Adaptation: "It" was adapted into a successful two-part film series, with the first part released in 2017 and the second in 2019.
Famous Dialogue: "We all float down here."

"The Stand" (1978):
Plot Synopsis: "The Stand" is an epic post-apocalyptic novel set in a world decimated by a deadly virus. It follows the journey of survivors, including Stu Redman and Frannie Goldsmith, as they align with either the forces of good or evil.
Movie Adaptation: "The Stand" has been adapted into a TV miniseries in 1994, and a new adaptation was announced for a limited series in 2020.
Famous Dialogue: "You can't spell 'pandemic' without 'panic.'"

"Misery" (1987):
Plot Synopsis: "Misery" focuses on Paul Sheldon, a novelist who becomes the captive of his obsessed fan, Annie Wilkes, after a car accident. Annie forces him to write a novel to her liking, and the story takes a dark and suspenseful turn.
Movie Adaptation: The novel was adapted into a successful film in 1990, starring James Caan and Kathy Bates, who won an Academy Award for her role.

Literature

CRASH COURSE IN
LITERATURE

AYN RAND

A PHILOSOPHER AND NOVELIST KNOWN FOR HER WORKS
OF OBJECTIVISM, WHICH EMPHASIZED INDIVIDUALISM
AND RATIONAL SELF-INTEREST.

Famous books with plot synopsis

"Atlas Shrugged" (Published in 1957):

Plot Synopsis:
"Atlas Shrugged" is a sweeping and philosophical novel set in a dystopian future America. The story unfolds as the country faces economic collapse due to increasing government regulations, collectivism, and the erosion of individual freedoms.

The narrative primarily follows the struggles of Dagny Taggart, a competent and visionary railroad executive, and Hank Rearden, an innovative steel industrialist, as they strive to maintain their businesses in the face of government interference and social decay.

As society deteriorates further, a mysterious figure known as John Galt leads a strike of the country's most productive individuals, who disappear and withdraw their talents from the world. Galt's strike aims to protest the exploitation of creative minds and the stifling of individual achievement.

The novel explores themes of capitalism, individualism, and the role of government, all while unraveling the mystery of who John Galt is and why he chose to lead this revolt.

"The Fountainhead" (Published in 1943):

Plot Synopsis:
"The Fountainhead" is a character-driven novel that revolves around the life of Howard Roark, a brilliant and uncompromising architect. Roark refuses to conform to architectural traditions and instead designs buildings according to his own innovative and individualistic principles.

The story explores Roark's journey as he faces opposition and rejection by architectural firms and traditionalists. His rival, Peter Keating, is the embodiment of conformity and popularity in the architectural world.

Roark's integrity and unwavering commitment to his vision lead to both professional success and personal conflicts, including his complex relationship with Dominique Francon, a fiercely independent woman who struggles to accept Roark's principles.

The novel delves into themes of individualism, integrity, and the creative process, as it challenges societal norms and celebrates the pursuit of one's own path.

Powerful Quotes from Ayn Rand

"Who is John Galt?" This recurring question becomes a symbol of resistance and individualism in the novel.

"I could die for you. But I couldn't, and wouldn't, live for you."

"I am. I think. I will."

"The question isn't who is going to let me; it's who is going to stop me."

"You can avoid reality, but you cannot avoid the consequences of avoiding reality."

"The creator stands on his own judgment. The parasite follows the opinions of others."

"I could have you arrested. But what for? Not for looting, but for being a looter who didn't loot enough."

"I owe nothing to my brothers, nor do I gather debts from them. I ask none to live for me, nor do I live for any others."

"My happiness needs no higher aim to vindicate it. My happiness is not the means to any end. It is the end. It is its own goal. It is its own purpose."

CRASH COURSE IN
LITERATURE

QUOTES

WORDS TO KNOW

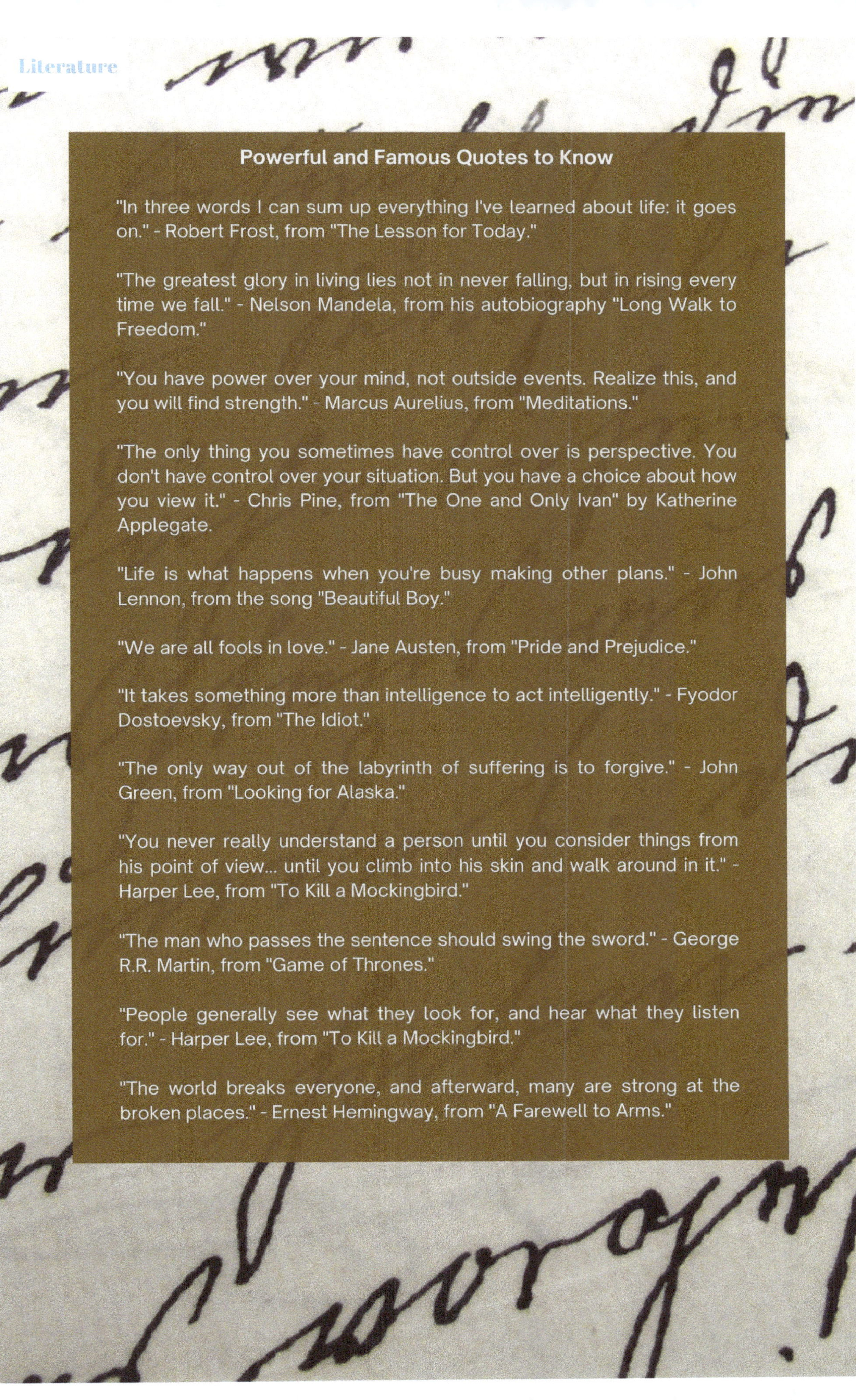

Powerful and Famous Quotes to Know

"In three words I can sum up everything I've learned about life: it goes on." - Robert Frost, from "The Lesson for Today."

"The greatest glory in living lies not in never falling, but in rising every time we fall." - Nelson Mandela, from his autobiography "Long Walk to Freedom."

"You have power over your mind, not outside events. Realize this, and you will find strength." - Marcus Aurelius, from "Meditations."

"The only thing you sometimes have control over is perspective. You don't have control over your situation. But you have a choice about how you view it." - Chris Pine, from "The One and Only Ivan" by Katherine Applegate.

"Life is what happens when you're busy making other plans." - John Lennon, from the song "Beautiful Boy."

"We are all fools in love." - Jane Austen, from "Pride and Prejudice."

"It takes something more than intelligence to act intelligently." - Fyodor Dostoevsky, from "The Idiot."

"The only way out of the labyrinth of suffering is to forgive." - John Green, from "Looking for Alaska."

"You never really understand a person until you consider things from his point of view... until you climb into his skin and walk around in it." - Harper Lee, from "To Kill a Mockingbird."

"The man who passes the sentence should swing the sword." - George R.R. Martin, from "Game of Thrones."

"People generally see what they look for, and hear what they listen for." - Harper Lee, from "To Kill a Mockingbird."

"The world breaks everyone, and afterward, many are strong at the broken places." - Ernest Hemingway, from "A Farewell to Arms."

Powerful and Famous Quotes to Know

"To be yourself in a world that is constantly trying to make you something else is the greatest accomplishment." - Ralph Waldo Emerson, from his essay "Self-Reliance."

"The only way to do great work is to love what you do." - Steve Jobs, from his Stanford University commencement speech.

"It is our choices, Harry, that show what we truly are, far more than our abilities." - J.K. Rowling, from "Harry Potter and the Chamber of Secrets."

"The only thing necessary for the triumph of evil is for good men to do nothing." - Edmund Burke, often attributed, from various writings.

"The unexamined life is not worth living." - Socrates, from Plato's "Apology."

"It is not the strongest of the species that survives, nor the most intelligent; it is the one most responsive to change." - Charles Darwin, from "The Origin of Species."

"The only limit to our realization of tomorrow will be our doubts of today." - Franklin D. Roosevelt, from various speeches.

"To be yourself in a world that is constantly trying to make you something else is the greatest accomplishment." - Ralph Waldo Emerson, from "Self-Reliance."

"The more that you read, the more things you will know. The more that you learn, the more places you'll go." - Dr. Seuss, from "I Can Read With My Eyes Shut!"

"It does not do to dwell on dreams and forget to live." - J.K. Rowling, from "Harry Potter and the Sorcerer's Stone."

"The only real prison is fear, and the only real freedom is freedom from fear." - Aung San Suu Kyi, from "Freedom from Fear."

"Do not go gentle into that good night. Rage, rage against the dying of the light." - Dylan Thomas, from his poem "Do Not Go Gentle into That Good Night."

CRASH COURSE IN
LITERATURE

Kafka

A German-speaking
Bohemian writer,
renowned for his surreal
and existential works
that often explore
themes of alienation,
bureaucracy, and
absurdity.

Famous works of Franz Kafka

"The Metamorphosis" (1915):

Gregor Samsa, a young man, wakes up one morning to find himself transformed into a giant insect. His physical transformation disrupts his life and his relationships with his family, who are repelled by his appearance.

The novella delves into the emotional and psychological effects of this bizarre transformation on Gregor and his family as they grapple with the grotesque and the absurd.

"The Trial" (1925):

Josef K., a young and seemingly innocent man, is arrested by unidentified authorities without being informed of his crime. He is caught up in a complex and surreal legal system.

The novel follows Josef K.'s attempts to navigate the bewildering bureaucracy and find out why he is on trial. It explores themes of guilt, powerlessness, and the arbitrary nature of justice.

"The Castle" (1926):

The novel revolves around K., a land surveyor who arrives in a remote village with the intention of working for the castle officials. However, he faces obstacles and struggles to gain access to the castle itself.

Throughout the narrative, K. encounters a host of eccentric characters and experiences the oppressive and labyrinthine bureaucracy of the castle. The story is left unfinished, adding to its enigmatic nature.

"A Hunger Artist" (1924):

This is a short story that focuses on a professional hunger artist who starves himself in public as a form of performance art. The story explores themes of isolation, the pursuit of artistic expression, and the indifference of the public.

"In the Penal Colony" (1919):

Set on a remote island, the story centers on an elaborate execution machine that carves the sentence of the condemned prisoner onto their body over the course of twelve hours.

The narrative follows a traveler's encounter with the prison's officer, who is a fervent believer in the machine and its torturous process. The story raises questions about justice, punishment, and cruelty.

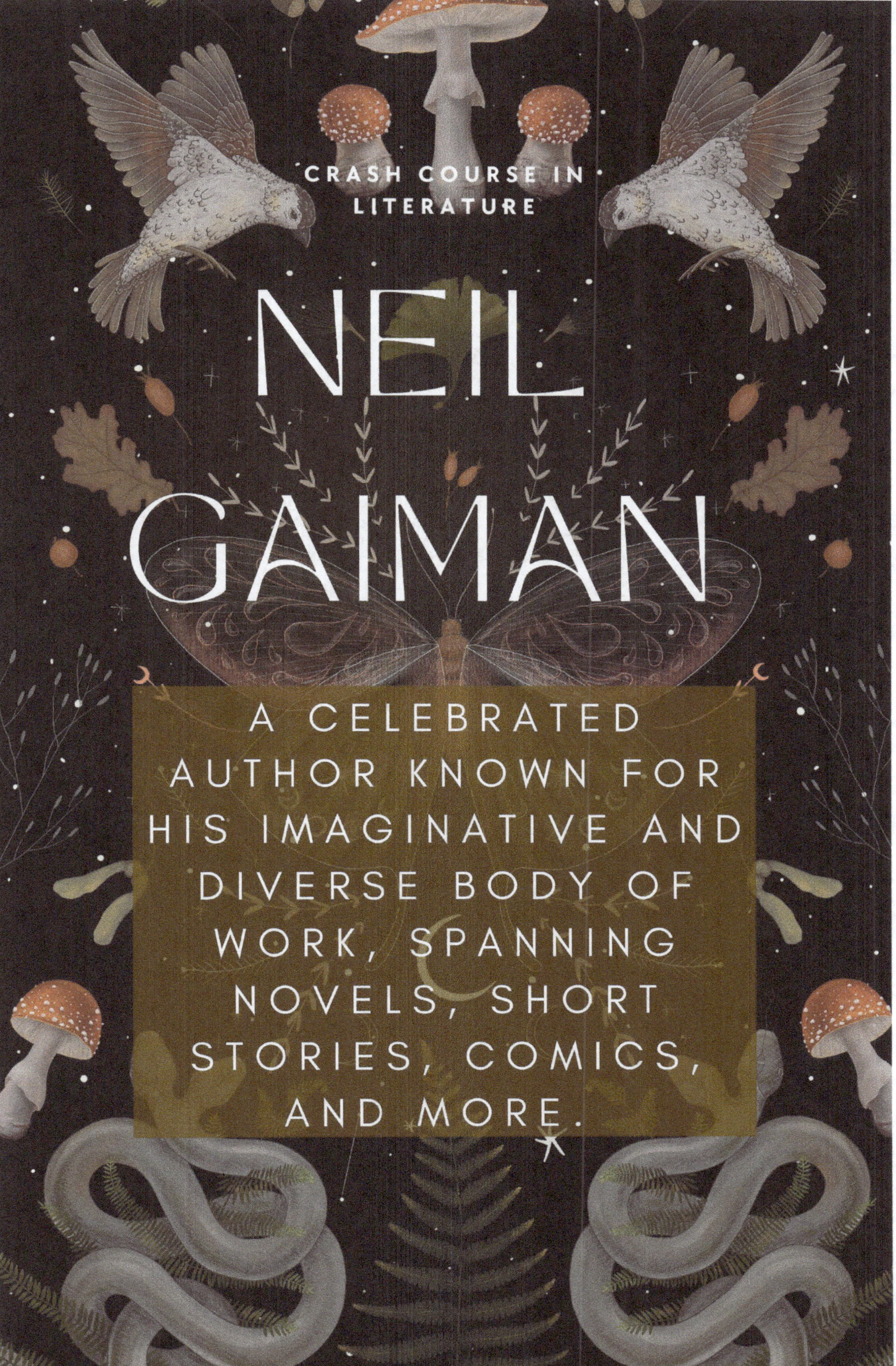
CRASH COURSE IN
LITERATURE

NEIL
GAIMAN

A CELEBRATED
AUTHOR KNOWN FOR
HIS IMAGINATIVE AND
DIVERSE BODY OF
WORK, SPANNING
NOVELS, SHORT
STORIES, COMICS,
AND MORE.

Famous works of Neil Gaiman

"American Gods" (2001):

In "American Gods," ex-convict Shadow Moon is released from prison only to discover that his wife has died in a car accident. On his journey home for her funeral, he encounters the enigmatic Mr. Wednesday, who offers him a job as his bodyguard. Shadow soon becomes embroiled in a conflict between ancient gods from various mythologies and new gods representing modern technology and media. The novel explores themes of belief, mythology, and the evolving American identity.

"Coraline" (2002):

"Coraline" is a dark fantasy novella about a young girl named Coraline Jones who discovers a hidden door in her new home that leads to an alternate reality. In this eerie otherworld, she finds an idealized version of her life but soon realizes that it hides sinister secrets. Coraline must confront a malevolent entity and rescue her real parents and other trapped souls.

"Neverwhere" (1996):

"Neverwhere" is a novel that blends urban fantasy with a hidden magical world. Richard Mayhew, a Londoner, helps a young woman named Door, who is bleeding and wounded on the streets. In doing so, he is drawn into London Below, a parallel city populated by fantastical characters and places. Richard embarks on a quest to uncover the truth about Door's family and the dark forces pursuing her.

"Good Omens" (co-written with Terry Pratchett, 1990):

"Good Omens" is a humorous and satirical novel that explores the end of the world. It follows the unlikely friendship between Aziraphale, an angel, and Crowley, a demon, who have grown fond of Earth and its inhabitants. When they learn that the apocalypse is imminent, they team up to prevent it and save humanity, leading to a series of comedic and otherworldly misadventures.

"The Sandman" (1989-1996, comic book series):

"The Sandman" is a critically acclaimed comic book series that follows Dream, one of the Endless, a group of powerful and immortal beings. Dream, also known as Morpheus, is the personification of dreams and storytelling. The series explores Dream's vast realm, the Dreaming, and his interactions with various mythological and supernatural characters.

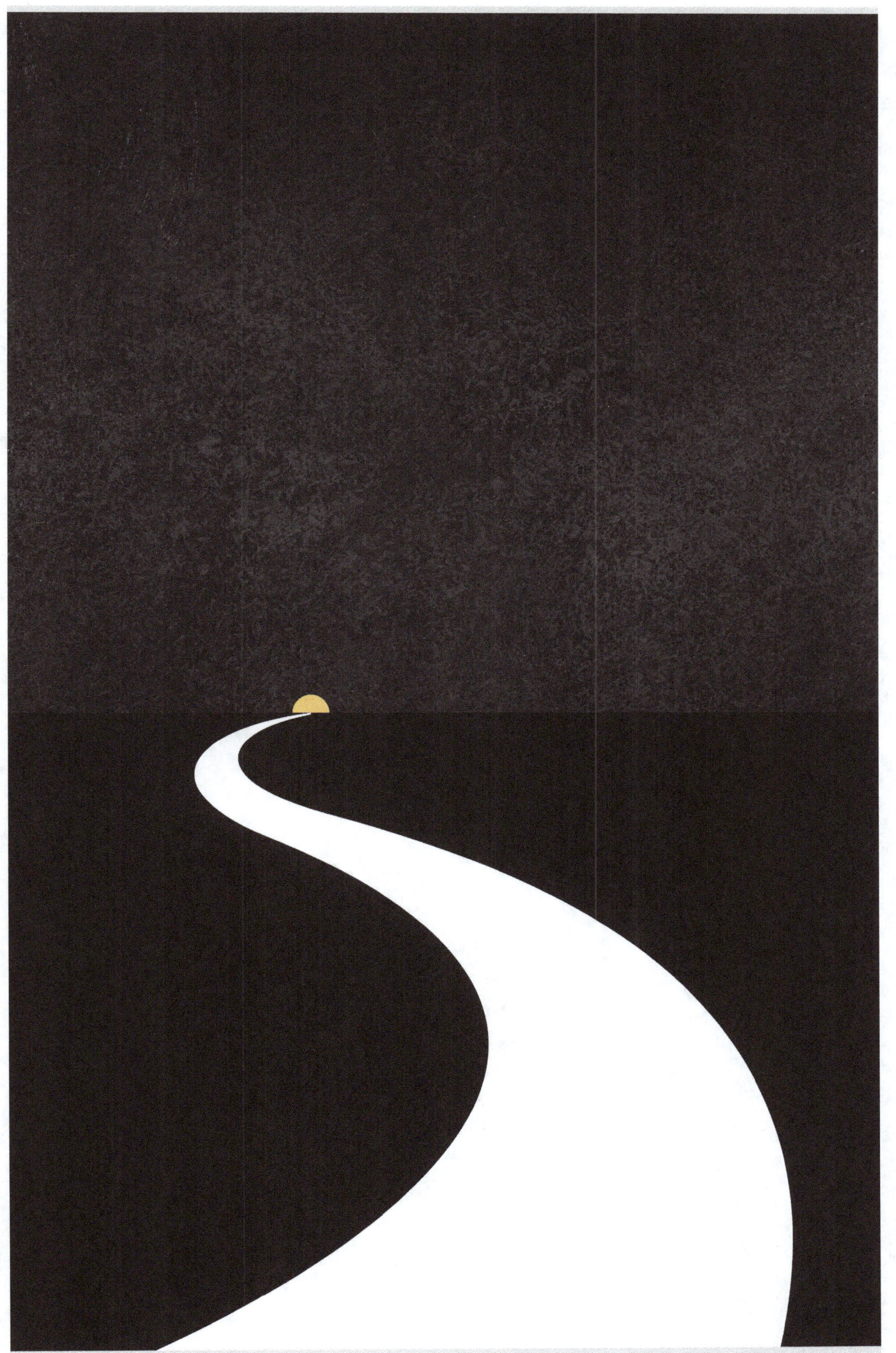

www.ingramcontent.com/pod-product-compliance
Lightning Source LLC
Chambersburg PA
CBHW080929260726
48661CB00010B/3853